Welcome!

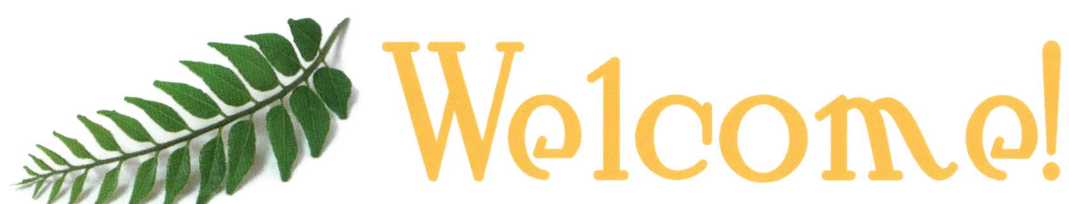

Welcome along on this Paleo/ AIP Indian Cooking Adventure! My name is Bethany Darwin and I'll be your guide on this journey through the flavors and kitchens of India. But, not to worry, as on any good adventure, I've done all the necessary preparation to assure that this journey is safe for all of our adventurers. Whether you have allergies or have chosen the paleo or AIP diets for health benefits, this cookbook will help guide you through the food culture of India and allow you to enjoy the flavors all while keeping you safe from grains, dairy, eggs, nuts, seeds and nightshades. So, hold on and keep your hands inside the tuk-tuk at all times and let's get on with this adventure!

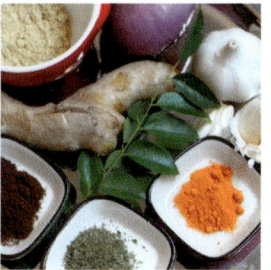 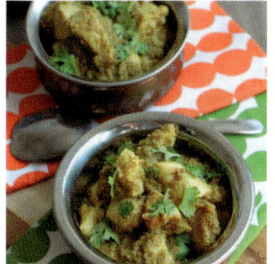 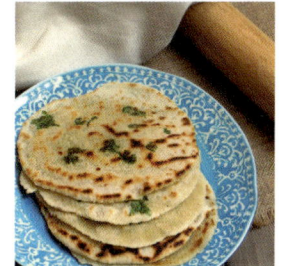 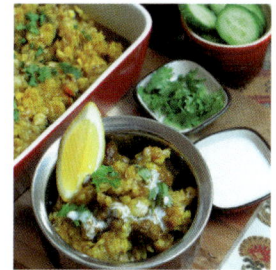 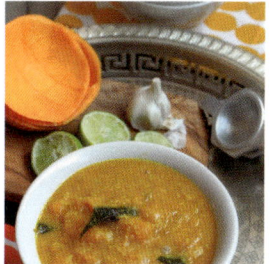

Dedication:

This book is dedicated to my supportive hubby, my "Darwing," Joseph.
Thanks for being my taste tester extraordinaire, for giving helpful feedback on recipes, for naming many of the dishes and for encouraging me to write this book.

To my mother-in-law, Kala, who has graciously learned to cook AIP and whose dinners are the inspiration for several of the recipes in this book.

To my mom (Judy), my grandmas (Sybil & Evelyn)
and all the other women who let me
make messes in their kitchen when I was a little girl
and taught me to love cooking.

And to my dad, Gary, who loves spicy food even more than I do.

Table of Contents

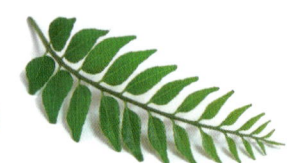

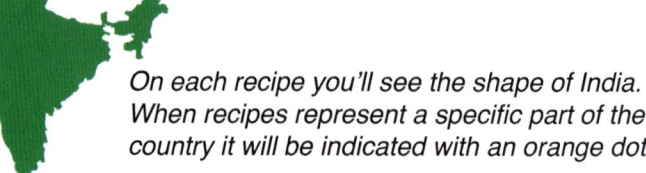

On each recipe you'll see the shape of India. When recipes represent a specific part of the country it will be indicated with an orange dot.

Introduction

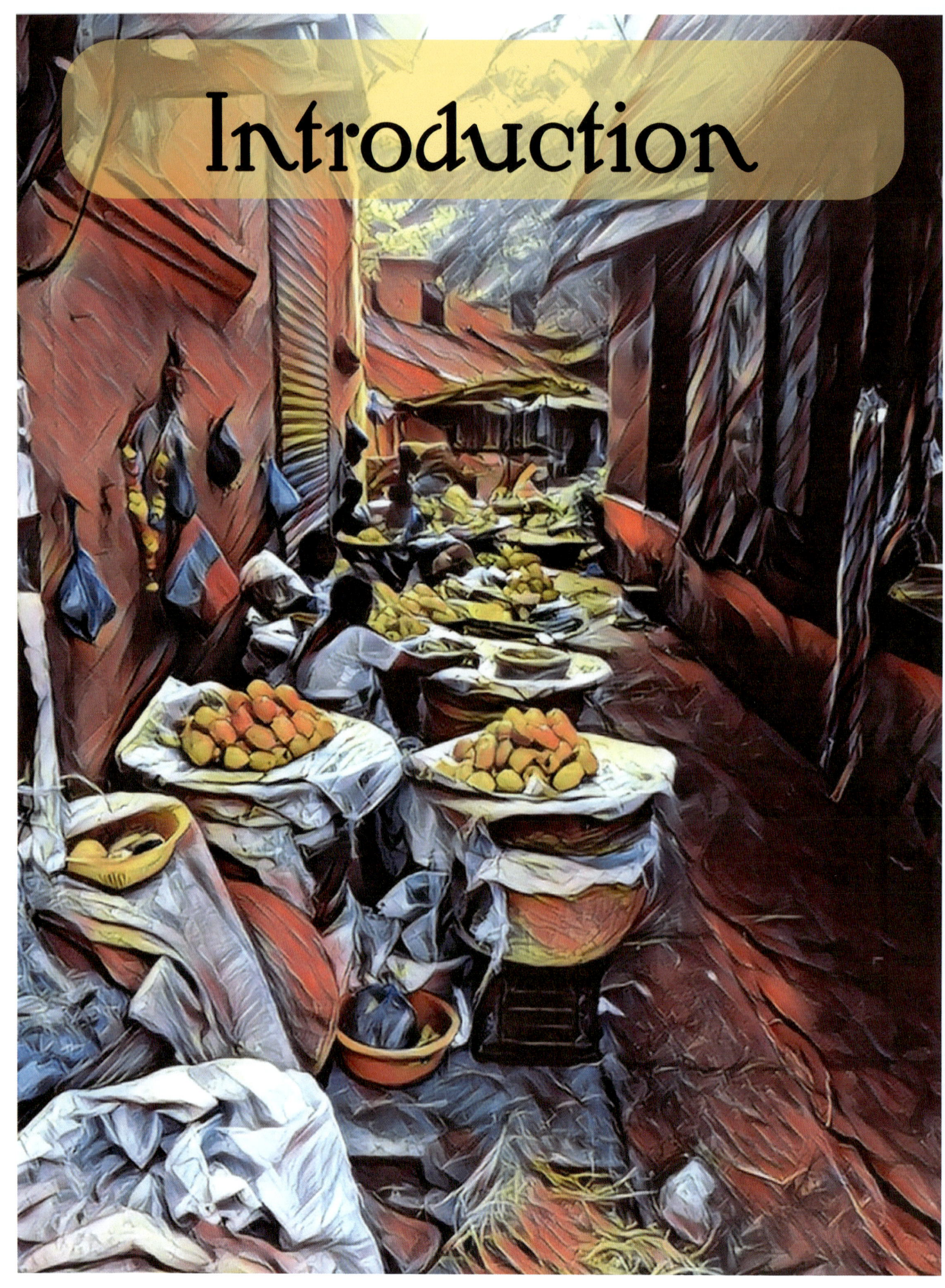

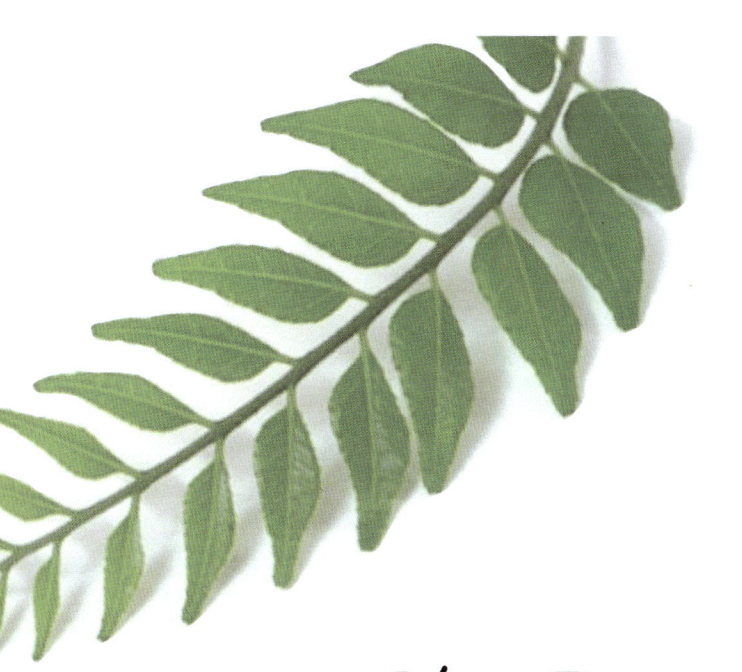

Grain Free
Dairy Free
Nightshade Free
Egg Free
Nut Free

My Paleo/ AIP
Indian
Adventure

60+ allergen friendly Indian recipes,
so you can enjoy Indian food again!

Bethany Darwin

All recipes were created and photographed
by Bethany Darwin

Disclaimer: Please note that the author is not a medical professional and that this cookbook is not intended to be medical advice. Please contact a medical professional before making any kind of dietary change.

What is AIP? What is Paleo?

What exactly is the Autoimmune Protocol (AIP)? There are many books and resources that answer this question, so I'm not going to recreate the wheel, but here are some of the answers I give people when they ask about my 'unusual' diet.

~ AIP is Paleo with a twist.

~ AIP is a low inflammation diet.

~ AIP is a nutrient dense way of eating.

~ AIP is a decision to eat vegetables, quality meats and seafood and some fruit.

Those answers are usually good enough to placate my friends (or strangers on the airplane), but if you're new to AIP, here are the BASICS. The autoimmune protocol is a diet template that removes high inflammation causing foods and replaces them with nutrient dense and gut healing foods. This healing protocol is designed to help people suffering from auto immune conditions to remove the inflammation from their bodies and relieve many of their auto immune related symptoms. AIP isn't a cure for auto immune disease, but is designed to help you figure out what triggers your flares and set you out on a healing journey.

The first thing that most people want to know when they get started on any sort of healing protocol (or any new diet plan) is 'what can't I eat?' I prefer to think of what I can eat and you'll see an AIP plate on page 7 showing all the wonderful foods that you can enjoy on AIP.

But first, here are the <u>FOODS that need to be AVOIDED</u> on the elimination phase of the AIP:

- · ALL Grains - wheat, corn, rice, quinoa, oats, etc.
- · ALL Dairy - milk, cheese, yogurt, ice cream, etc.
- · ALL Nuts and Seeds - this includes nut milks, nut flours, nut oils and seed based spices
- · Nightshade Vegetables - potatoes, tomatoes, eggplant, all peppers (sweet and hot peppers), tomatillos, paprika (other chili based spices)
- · Eggs
- · Legumes - beans, lentils, peanuts, soy (all soy based products)
- · Coffee

- Chocolate
- Refined sugars
- Modern vegetable oils
- ALL processed foods - all emulsifiers, thickeners and food additives
- Black pepper
- Alcohol

The key behind the AIP diet is that it's not just a list of foods to remove from your life. It's also about the addition of nutrient dense foods. AIP meals are comprised mainly of vegetables along with grass fed meats, seafood, offal, and bone broth. See the 'plate' on the next page for a visual look at what makes up the AIP diet. Notice how great a role vegetables play.

So, what can you eat on the AIP Paleo Diet? You can enjoy all cuts of meat, poultry and seafood. You can enjoy all vegetables with the exception of those in the nightshade family. You can enjoy all fruits (with the exception of nightshade fruits again). You can enjoy a variety of herbs and seasonings as well as some extras that you'll notice on the next page. And, most importantly, you can enjoy the feeling of eating well to help your body and hopefully enjoy relief from pain and healing from inflammation.

Another thing to keep in mind at the start is that the AIP (at least in it's strictest elimination phase) isn't meant to last forever. The plan is designed to follow the elimination phase diet until you feel relief from your AI symptoms and then systematically reintroduce foods. For more information on reintroductions, please see page 103.

A Note on Treats:

Although there are 'treats' in this book and they are made with AIP compliant ingredients, this doesn't make them a typical part of the AIP diet. Treats are just what they sound like - *a special food reserved for occasional consumption and special occasions*. This is especially true of the Indian treats in this book. They are all 100% AIP compliant, but they are still high in natural sugars and will still cause inflammation in your body, so go easy on them.

What's on my AIP Plate?

Fruit: Limited to 20 gr. of fructose a day

Offal: liver, kidney, heart, etc. 3-5x a week

Grass Fed or Pasture Raised Meats + Seafoods: Beef, lamb, pork, bison, venison, chicken, turkey, duck, fish, shrimp, mussels, crab, etc. Seafood should be eaten 3x a week.

Healthy Fats: coconut oil, avocado oil, olive oil, palm shortening, lard & other animal fats

Vegetables: The AIP diet is vegetable dense. Fill your menu up with a variety of vegetables. Try to get 8-14 cups of vegetables a day - Green vegetables, colorful vegetables, starchy vegetables, cruciferous vegetables, sea vegetables.

All vegetables are compliant except nightshades.

Extras...

Seasonings -
- pink himalayan salt
- aromatics like ginger and garlic
- fresh and dried herbs
- non-seed-based spices (cinnamon, cloves, saffron, turmeric & mace)
- vinegars (apple cider, balsamic & wine vinegars)
- coconut aminos
- sweeteners in moderation (honey, molasses, maple syrup, dates)
- coconut products in moderation
- carob

Probiotic foods - fermented vegetables, kombucha, etc.

Glycine-rich Foods - like bone broth, gelatin, collagen

Teas - Black, green & rooibos in moderation

India and Indian Food

India is the 7th largest country in the world by area and and has the 2nd highest population in the world with 1.2 billion residents, divided into 29 states. Needless to say, India is a vast and diverse country. This diversity comes out in every way from language to culture to clothes to religion... and for the sake of foodies like us.... to food.

What do you think of when you think of Indian food? Butter chicken? Chicken Tikka? Biryani? Or maybe all you know of Indian food is a non-specific *curry*.

Indian food is so much more than these well known dishes. In the same way that Mexican food is more than tacos and American food is more than hot dogs and fries. In the following pages we're going to explore traditional Indian foods and how they can be adapted to fit into the AIP template.

The food of India is as varied and diverse as the country itself. It's true that around the country you'll find similarities in cuisine, like a reliance on rice and chili, but each of the twenty-nine states is known for specific dishes. Some of these key dishes and the state they are from are:
• Kashmir - Rogan Josh - pg. 48
• Tamil Nadu - Chicken Chettinad Curry - pg. 63
• Kerala - Fish Molee - pg. 71
• Andhra Pradesh - Hyderabadi Biriyani - pg. 53
• Haryana - Gajar Methi - pg. 84
• Goa - Fish and Mango Curry - pg. 70

In the southern coastal states of Kerala, Tamil Nadu, and Goa, the cuisine is heavy on coconut, tropical fruits and seafood. Although these dishes are often still full of heat from chili peppers, their flavor is aromatic and tropical with curry leaves, ginger, garlic, onions and coconut forming the base of many of the dishes. These are the dishes you can enjoy on a hot and humid summer afternoon while sipping a Jal Jeera (pg. 90).

Whereas in the far north of India, in the states of Kashmir and Punjab you'll find heavier meat and veggie based dishes. These parts of the country have hard winters and residents need the warmth of comfort foods. These dishes often add the flavors one might associate with fall (cinnamon, mace, cloves) to add depth to their recipes, along with the prevailing heat from the infamous red chili.

Interesting note, the red chili pepper actually isn't actually native to India. Chili peppers are actually native to Mexico where they have been cultivated since 3500 BC. They only became part of Indian cuisine after Christopher Columbus' *navigational error*. He had set out for India in search of pepper (black pepper), but instead found the red chili in central America and brought it back to Europe giving it the name 'pepper.' Shortly thereafter, the chili made it's way into the hearts and kitchens of Indians and now it's almost impossible to think of Indian cuisine without this bright little nightshade that packs such a punch.

And, as the story goes, one of the reasons that chili peppers ands spice became so important in India was because of the quality of river water in cities like delhi. The theory was that the spice would be so intense that they'd need to cut the heat with a generous portion of ghee and the two combined would help to combat the gut issues that come along with drinking dirty water.

While we're talking about food, it should also be noted that much of the food culture of India is defined by religion. 80% of Indians are Hindu and as a rule, Hindus never eat beef as they esteem the cow. And, many Hindus are complete vegetarians, deriving their protein from legumes, nuts, yogurt, ghee and paneer (a soft cheese). Almost 14% of Indians are Muslim and they don't eat pork. The remaining 6% is made up of other religions - Christianity, Catholicism, Jainism, Buddhism and Sikhism. Sikhs eat a simple vegetarian diet while Buddhists eat a vegan diet and Jains eat an egg-free vegetarian diet that also excludes all root vegetables because to consume them you must kill the whole plant, while other vegetables you leave the plant and only remove the portion to be eaten.

Looking into the food culture of India, is like going on an exploration through the history of this diverse land. Regional dishes may seem to simply be a part of life, but you dig a little deeper and you'll discover how this particular dish has evolved over the years based on population migration and flavor imports from around the world and you'll see the Indian influence in the food cultures of the rest of the world... chicken tikka masala is now listed as the national dish of England.

But, sadly for all of us following the AIP diet and lifestyle, Indian food is almost always characterized by nightshades and seed based spices. How does one take these amazing dishes of India and turn them into something that can be both eaten and enjoyed by all without a hint of nightshades?

Well, it was a bit of a challenge, but with the help of my ever supportive hubby (who happens to be from Tamil Nadu), I've reworked as many of these traditional recipes as possible to remove the offending nightshades and seed based spices as well as dairy and grains and believe that what I have for you is a collection of Indian recipes that you and your family will be able to enjoy for years to come.

The important thing to keep in mind at the start of this journey is that Indian food (for the most part), is simple, home style dishes that are rich and full of deep flavor, and packed with the produce that's locally grown and readily available. That's one of the reasons for the variety of recipes around the country. In the southern coastal areas where coconut palms are everywhere, the flavor of curries are developed through the use of fresh coconut meat, whereas in the north you'll find more cream and yogurt used to give dishes their creamy goodness.

Through this book, we're going to explore to flavors of India and do so in a way that's safe for all of us on the adventure we call AIP. And my hope is that you'll take the ideas in these recipes and make them your own, creating your own spin on Indian food

NOTES:
- **meat** - Much of India is Hindu and vegetarian, and even for those who would be willing to eat it, beef is not easily available in India. In this book, you'll find many lamb recipes as lamb, mutton and goat are commonly available in India. Any of these lamb dishes could easily be substituted with beef or venison.
- **spices** - All the recipes in this book are written to be 100% AIP compliant. Many recipes include a reintroduction note to help you know which spices to add once you have been able to successfully reintroduce seed based spices. Very few reintroduction notes will be given for nightshades as I am unable to test them for you.

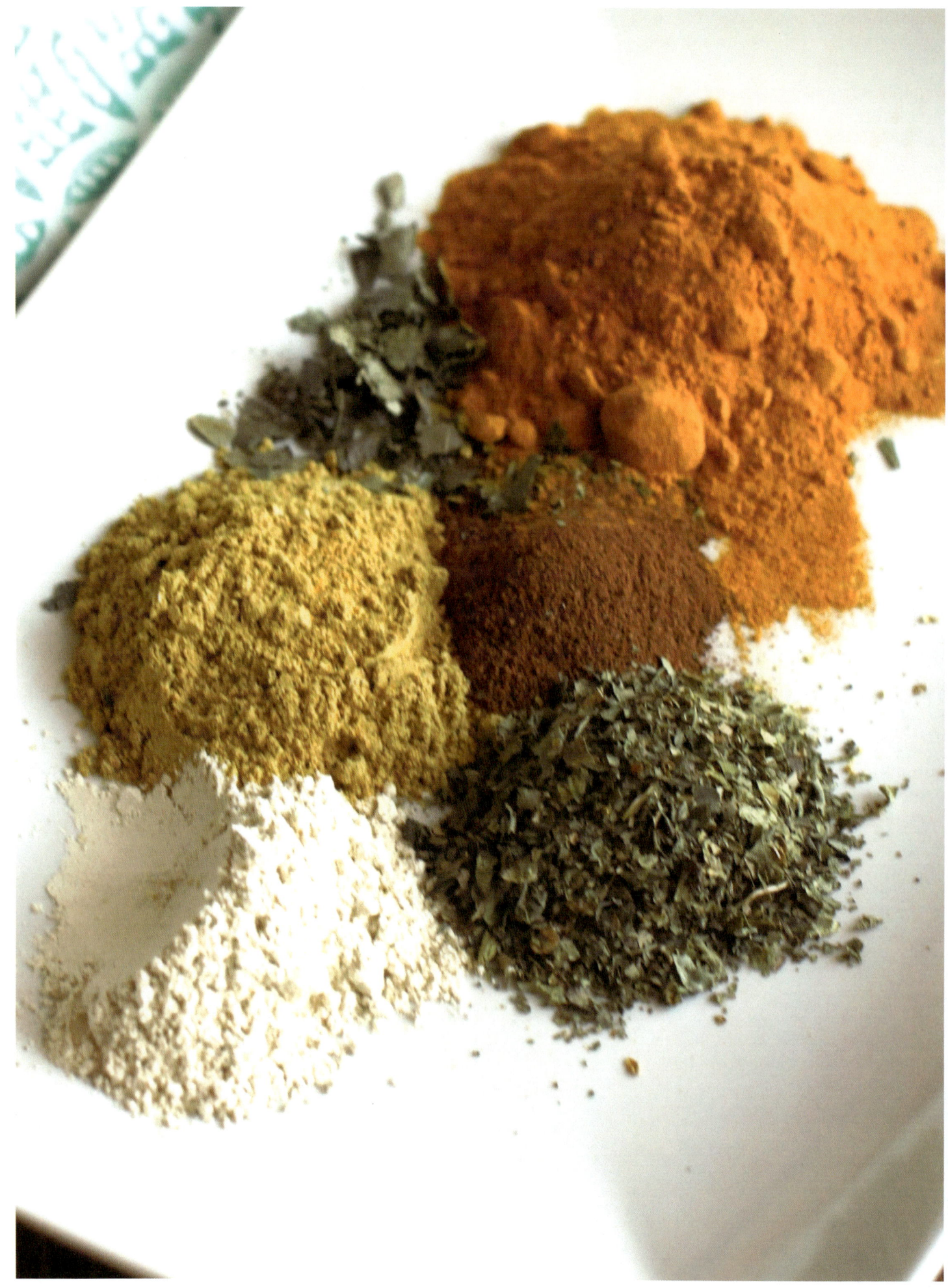

Grieving and Reclaiming Spice on the Autoimmune Protocol

This book is a labor of love as I continue to process through the absence of "true" (or maybe I should say traditional) Indian foods and the heat and spice that comes with them. So, as we get started on this Paleo/ AIP Indian adventure together, I want to share something a little more personal in nature with you. I think this will resonate with many of you.

For much of my life I have suffered with undiagnosed back pain. Then, about 8 years ago I started having eye pain and was diagnosed with an AI condition called uveitis. My awesome eye doctor convinced me after the 2nd flare that this condition is often related to other AI conditions and sent me for testing and sure enough, the back pain was explained with the diagnosis of spodylarthritis. My rheumatologist started talking all kinds of scary drug treatments and I freaked out and googled *diet for autoimmune disease* and found 'the paleo mom.' I read about the diet and jumped right in within a few days and haven't looked back. After 3 months I was completely off all anti-inflammatories and pain meds and felt like a new woman. I couldn't believe how great it felt to sleep all night and wake up pain free.

In the 3+ years that I've been following AIP, I've made a few reintroductions.... eggs, seed spices, and the occasional serving of white rice, square of dark chocolate or white potato. I try to keep most of my reintros for traveling or eating out and stay mostly compliant at home. I haven't actually tried reintroducing any nightshades other than the occasional potato because when I accidentally eat some I react pretty quickly and honestly I've gotten used to life without them.

Before AIP I loved spicy foods... Indian, Thai, Mexican, etc. I always had a bottle of tabasco sauce with me and used it to top many of my meals. There was no such thing as a bland meal in my home. And, I believed that's how life should be lived.

And then came AIP and the realization that nightshades (especially chili peppers) were not my friend. In fact, a thai green curry was my last meal before AIP and the one that pushed me over the edge and convinced me that it was time to start this journey. As I began AIP and cut nightshades out of my life, I literally went through the five stages of grief.

- Denial - *I've eaten spicy food my whole life, a little bit won't hurt me.... This is something other people are dealing with, I'm fine with peppers.*

- Anger - *This isn't fair.... I'll never be able to eat out again... I just want to be like everyone else and eat a bowl of curry.*

- Bargaining - *I'll give up everything else and I'll be able to keep nightshade spices.... I'll never eat chocolate again if I can just enjoy a good biryani.*

- 🌿 **Depression** - *I guess all my food will have to be boring and bland.... Why even try cooking if I can't enjoy spicy chili and curry.*
- 🌿 **Acceptance** - *Ginger and daikon and cilantro and turmeric are my new best friends.... I may not be able to recreate perfectly authentic flavors, but I can get some heat and depth of flavor and it tastes like Indian food.... My food tastes good again!*

How about you? Did you go through those same stages and struggle as much about giving up chili peppers as I did? Or maybe your struggle was about coffee or chocolate or fill in the blank.

This is normal. This is how we, as humans, deal with loss (even with the seemingly simple loss of a favorite food). But, the point of the five stages of grief is that you're meant to work through them and come out on the other side.

Funnily enough, because this is also how life works, not long after coming to a point of accepting my new style of *Indian* cuisine and being pleased with it myself, an Indian man walked into my life. I started noticing this man more and more around church and in our small group and was enjoying getting to know him. But, there was a little voice in the back of my head that kept planting seeds of doubt.... *you can't eat Indian food... you wouldn't be able to cook his favorite foods.... it would be too much to ask him to live without 'his' food.*

But, these moments of doubt pointed me to my insufficiency to do anything on my own and how even though none of this made sense to me that it all made perfect sense to God.

Fast forward a few months from the time of those doubts and in God's perfect timing, this amazing man and I were married in April 2017. And guess what...

- he's ok with the fact that I won't be able to cook his favorite foods...
- he likes my AIP Indian foods... his favorites are Chicken Reshmi Kebabs and Prawn Masala.
- he wants to help me create more AIP Indian foods.... in fact, this book was his idea and couldn't have been written without him.

So, where are you on your spice grief journey?

Are you still at the point where you think it can't be done?

Have you resigned yourself to plain baked chicken and broccoli because you're afraid of all things spice?

Are you just constantly unsure about what spices and herbs are and aren't AIP compliant?

To make sure, we all know which spices are and aren't AIP friendly, please see the chart on the following page to make sure you never again have a bland or boring dish. Spice that baby up!

AIP Herbs & Spices

The basic rule of thumb for spices on the AIP is no nightshade spices (anything made from chili peppers) and no seed based spices. Fruit based spices (like black pepper) are also on the NO list during the elimination phase. Following is a list of herbs and spices that are YES for all stages of the AIP diet.

Aromatic Vegetables

- Chives
- Garlic
- Ginger root
- Horseradish
- Onions
- Onion Powder
- Shallots
- Turmeric root

Herbs

- Basil
- Bay leaves
- Chamomile
- Chervil
- Cilantro (Coriander leaf)
- Curry leaves
- Dill weed
- Fennel leaf
- Fenugreek leaves
- Kaffir lime leaves
- Lavender
- Lemon Balm
- Lemongrass
- Marjoram
- Oregano
- Parsley

- Peppermint
- Rosemary
- Sage
- Savory Leaves
- Tarragon
- Thyme

Spices

- Amchur Powder
- Asafetida
- Cinnamon
- Cloves
- Ginger powder
- Mace
- Pink Himalayan Salt
- Saffron
- Sea Salt
- Turmeric powder

Other Seasonings

- Apple cider vinegar
- Balsamic vinegar
- Coconut aminos
- Fish sauce
- Vanilla (alcohol free)
- Wasabi (additive free)

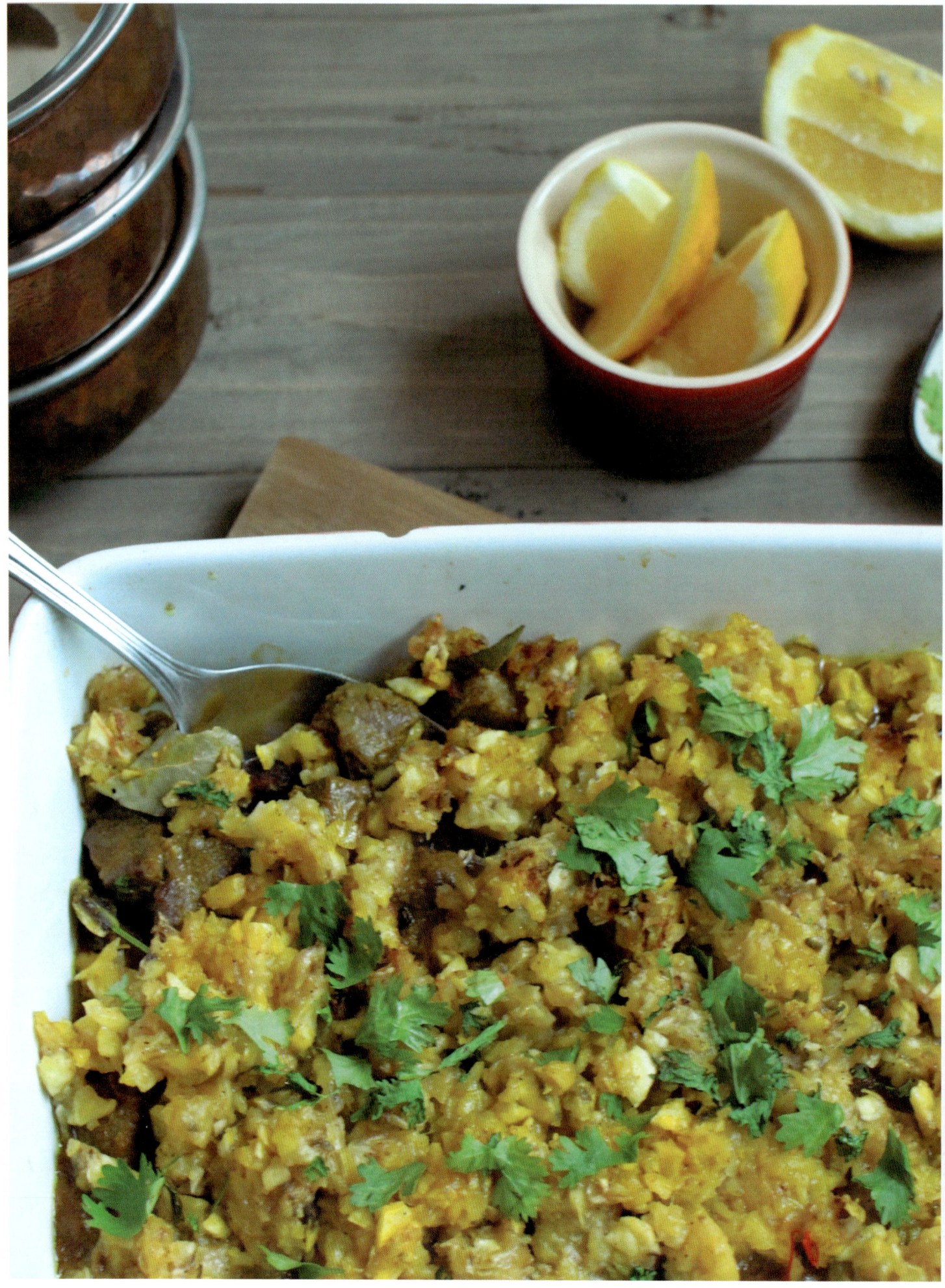

Glossary: Indian Cooking

- **Amchur Powder** - unripe green mango powder. Adds a citrusy/ tart taste to dishes and can be used where you might use a splash of lemon juice.
- **Asafetida** - the resin of a plant similar to fennel. Sometimes labeled by it's Hindi name (hing). It adds an umami flavor like onions and garlic and a depth of flavor. Watch out for extra ingredients.
- **Braising** - a method of cooking where food is seared at a high heat and then allowed to slow cook in a liquid or sauce. This is common in many curries as onions and spices are fried, meat is seared and then liquids are added and the lid is put on the pot to allow the meat to cook slowly and the flavors to infuse.
- **Cassava** - this root vegetable is also known as tapioca in some parts of the world, is grown in India and common in many dishes in it's own right. In AIP Indian cooking, cassava will sometimes be boiled to replace potatoes and other times it will be dried and ground and become the flour to replace both rice flour and wheat flour which are both common in Indian cooking.
- **Cilantro** - the leaf of the coriander plant, called coriander leaves in much of the world. These leaves add a spicy and citrusy flavor to foods and are popular in many Asian and Latin American cuisines. It is a polarizing herb that some people absolutely love and others just can't stand. Which camp are you in?
- **Cinnamon** - a spice derived from the inner bark of a family of trees that are native to south east asia. It is common in both sweet and savory dishes. Ground cinnamon powder is often added to recipes and cinnamon sticks are often cooked along with other whole spices at the beginning of the cooking process to infuse the oil (and therefore the whole dish) with their flavor. A 2 inch piece of cinnamon bark can be replaced with about 1/2 teaspoon of ground cinnamon.
- **Cloves** - aromatic flower buds that add a hint of sweetness and a warmth and depth of flavor to both sweet and savory dishes. They also have a lot of medicinal uses in India, including tooth pain relief. If you need to use ground cloves, 3 cloves is the same as 1/4 teaspoon ground cloves.
- **Coriander** - can refer to the fresh leaves (cilantro - which is AIP) or coriander seeds (which are not AIP, but are a stage 1 reintroduction as they are seed spices). Coriander seeds are common in Indian cooking and add a warm, almost spicy, flavor profile to foods.
- **Curry Leaves** - not to be confused with curry powder (which is actually a blend of spices), these leaves are very popular in South Indian and Sri Lankan cuisine. The tree is in the same family as citrus fruit trees and therefore the leaves add an aromatic flavor to dishes. Fresh curry leaves give the best flavor and can be stored in the freezer to extend their freshness, or you can use dry if you can't get fresh.
- **Fenugreek** - known as 'methi' in Indian cooking, both the seeds and leaves are common staples in an Indian kitchen. The seeds (non- AIP) and the leaves both have a complex sweet, bitter and savory flavor with almost a hint of maple. Fresh fenugreek leaves are often picked as microgreens and used in salads and other vegetable dishes.
- **Garam Masala** - a blend of spices commonly found in Indian and other south Asian cuisine. The word garam means to heat as the spices typically used in garam masala are know to raise body temperature. The typical blend consists of black pepper, white pepper, cloves, cinnamon, mace, bay leaf, cumin, coriander, black and green cardamon. It's important to note that every family has their own garam

masala mixture and that their recipes are often guarded as family secrets passed down from one generation to the next.

- **Ginger** - the root of a flowering plant that is used both fresh and dried to add heat to recipes. It is common in many cuisines. You'll find fresh ginger as the base of many Indian curries whereas pickled ginger is common in Japanese fare. Often in recipes, ginger root amount is measured as 1 inch or 2 inches... this refers to how much of the root you'll need to add to the dish. To peel fresh ginger root, you can scrape it with the back of a spoon. Peeled ginger root can be store in the freezer and then grated into your dish if you don't always have access to fresh. Dried ginger is much more concentrated in flavor, so use 1/4 teaspoon for every Tablespoon (or 1 inch piece) of fresh ginger called for.

- **Mace** - part of the nutmeg plant (NOTE- mace is AIP, while nutmeg is not) and is common in Northern Indian cooking. It has a subtle sweet flavor with hints of cinnamon, nutmeg and coriander and can often replace coriander seed (which isn't AIP) in your savory dishes.

- **Pink Himalayan Salt** - rock salt from the Punjab region of Pakistan, (not actually from the Himalayas). It has a slightly higher mineral concentration than other salts and therefore adds a deeper flavor to foods along with the saltiness.

- **Plantain** - otherwise known as cooking bananas and can be used at any stage of ripening. Green plantains are higher in starch content and can be used in similar preparations as potatoes (boiled, roasted, fried) and can be riced (see the Biryani recipe on pg. 53) to replace grains. While ripe plantains (yellow and turning black) are sweeter and great for dessert applications

- **Pomegranate** - the seeds (actually called arils) are the edible part of this fruit that originates from Iran to India. Although seeds aren't allowed on the AIP, pomegranate arils are AIP compliant and add a sweet and tangy taste to dishes. They're fun to toss in a salad or to use to top a biryani or curry for a pop of sweetness.

- **Saffron**- a spice derived from the crocus flower and is known as the most expensive spice in the world because of the challenge in harvesting. There are only 3 stigmas in each flower and they have to be harvested by hand. It adds the bright yellow color to many Indian dishes along with a subtle floral, honey like flavor that can't be replicated.

- **Tandoor** - a circular clay oven that's traditionally used in the north of India for things like naan bread.

- **Tamarind** - a pod like fruit common in south Indian cuisine. It has a sour sweet taste. It derives it's name from arab traders who referred to it as the Indian date. Tamarind paste can be bought in most asian and latin american grocers.

- **Tempering -** the cooking of whole spices and aromatics (like ginger, chili and curry leaves) briefly in hot oil to allow them to release their oils. Tempering either happens at the beginning of the cooking process as the base for a curry or biryani, or spices are tempered and then used to top completed dishes right before serving.

- **Turmeric** - comes from the underground stem of a plant in the ginger family and looks similar to ginger root, although it is smaller and has a darker skin and bright orange interior. You can use fresh of dried turmeric. It adds a bitter note to Indian dishes and is often used in combination with ginger, garlic, cinnamon, mace and coriander to produce a full flavor. It, like saffron, also adds a bright yellow color to food. And, it's known to have some anti-inflammatory properties.

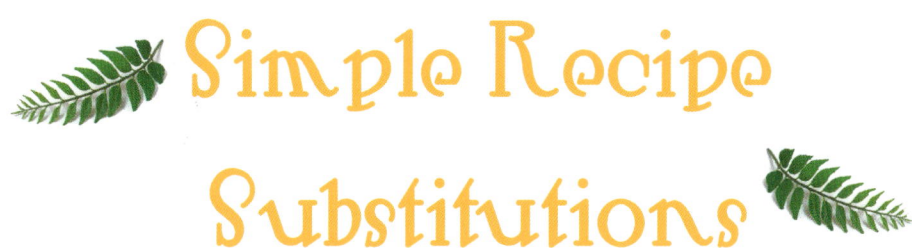

Simple Recipe Substitutions

When it comes to spice on the AIP, it can sometimes feel as if you need to be a master magician. But I'm going to let you behind the curtain and into the secret compartment in the hat to discover how you too can become a master of cooking with spice on the AIP diet. The trick is to understand why each spice is used. On the previous two pages (pg. 17 &18) you'll find a glossary of spices and other ingredients commonly found in Indian cooking along with a description of the spice, it's flavor and it's use. Once you know that ginger lends heat and mace has a subtle sweet and savory flavor you can start to see how they might be used to replace non-AIP spices in your favorite recipe.

Full disclosure: Nothing will perfectly mimic the 'my throat is on fire' flavor of a curry packed with red chili, but by following these simple substitutions you'll come to a point where you enjoy Indian cooking once more.

Here are a few simple ideas for recipe substitutions:
- when substituting dried herbs for fresh, use 1/3 the amount called for: 1 TBSP fresh herb = 1 tsp dried herb
- when substituting ground dried herbs for dried leaf herbs, use 1/2 the amount: 1 tsp dried leaf herb = 1/2 tsp ground dried herb
- when a recipe calls for **cinnamon** stick, use 1/2 tsp ground cinnamon instead of a 2 inch stick
- when a recipe calls for 1 tsp **allspice**, you can substitute 1/2 tsp cinnamon, 1/4 tsp mace & 1/8 tsp cloves
- when a recipe calls for 1 tsp ground **cardamon**, you can substitute 3/4 tsp ginger & 1/8 tsp cinnamon
- when a recipe calls for 1 tsp **cumin**, you can substitute 3/4 tsp ginger, 1/4 tsp mace & a couple of curry leaves
- when a recipe calls for 1 tsp **nutmeg**, you can substitute 1/2 tsp each of cinnamon and mace
- when a recipe calls for **chili** powder or fresh chili, you can increase the ginger or add some fresh grated radishes to the mix
- when a recipe calls for **tomatoes** you need to replace a sweet, savory and tangy flavor, so try a mix of pumpkin or carrot puree, a couple of fresh cranberries and a squeeze of lemon juice

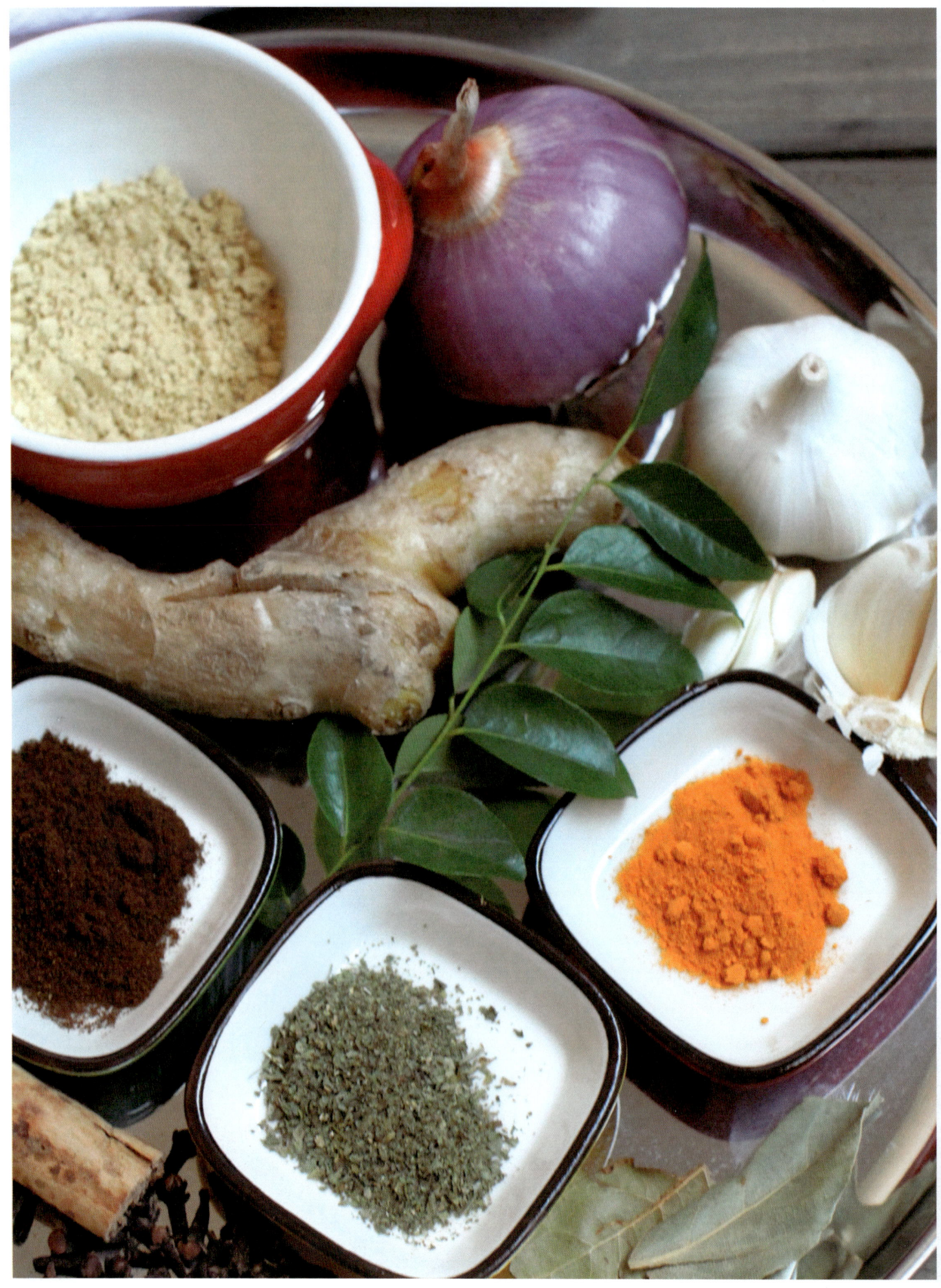

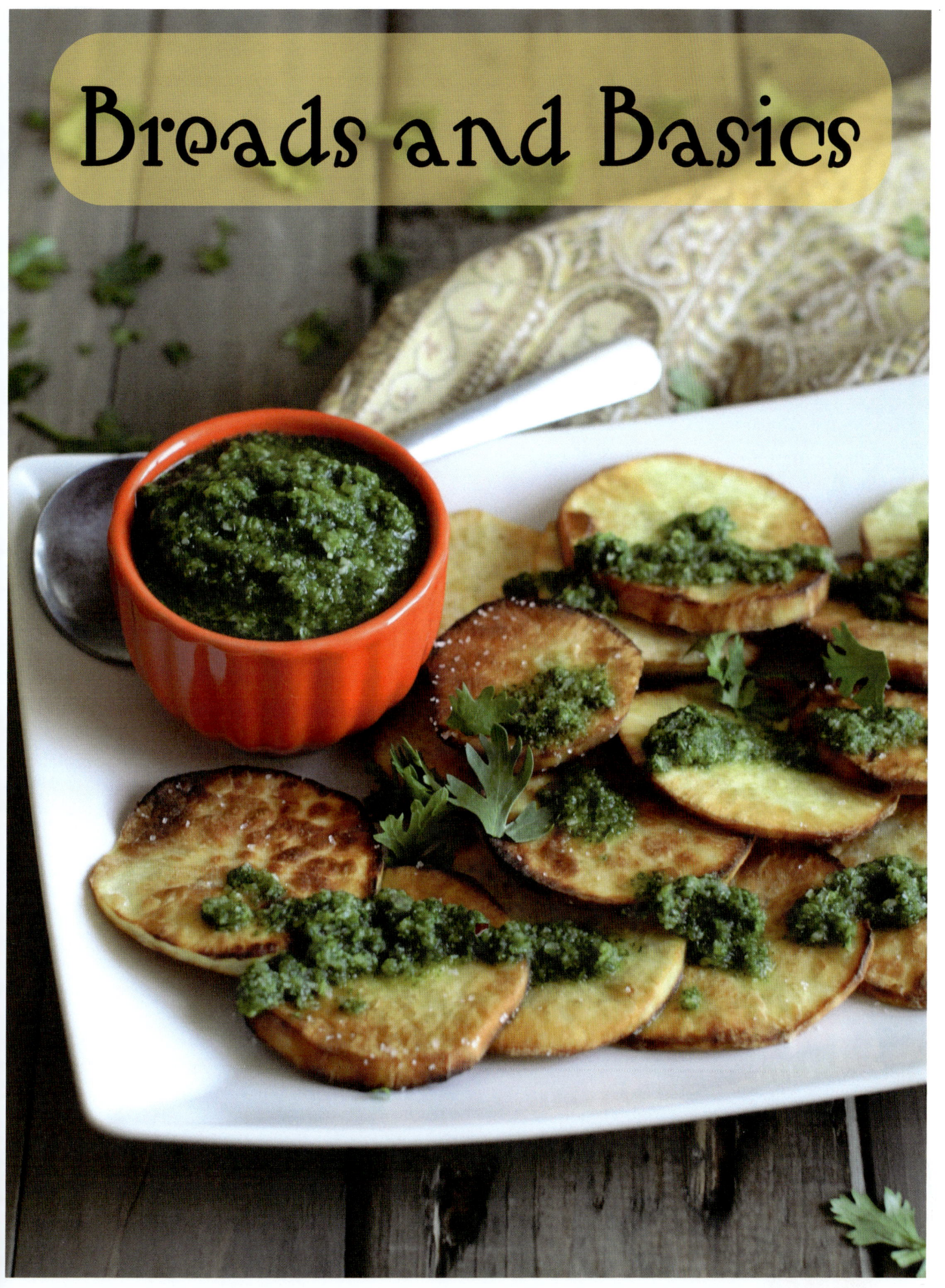

Breads and Basics

Garlic Coriander
Roti

Makes: 6   Time: 45 minutes

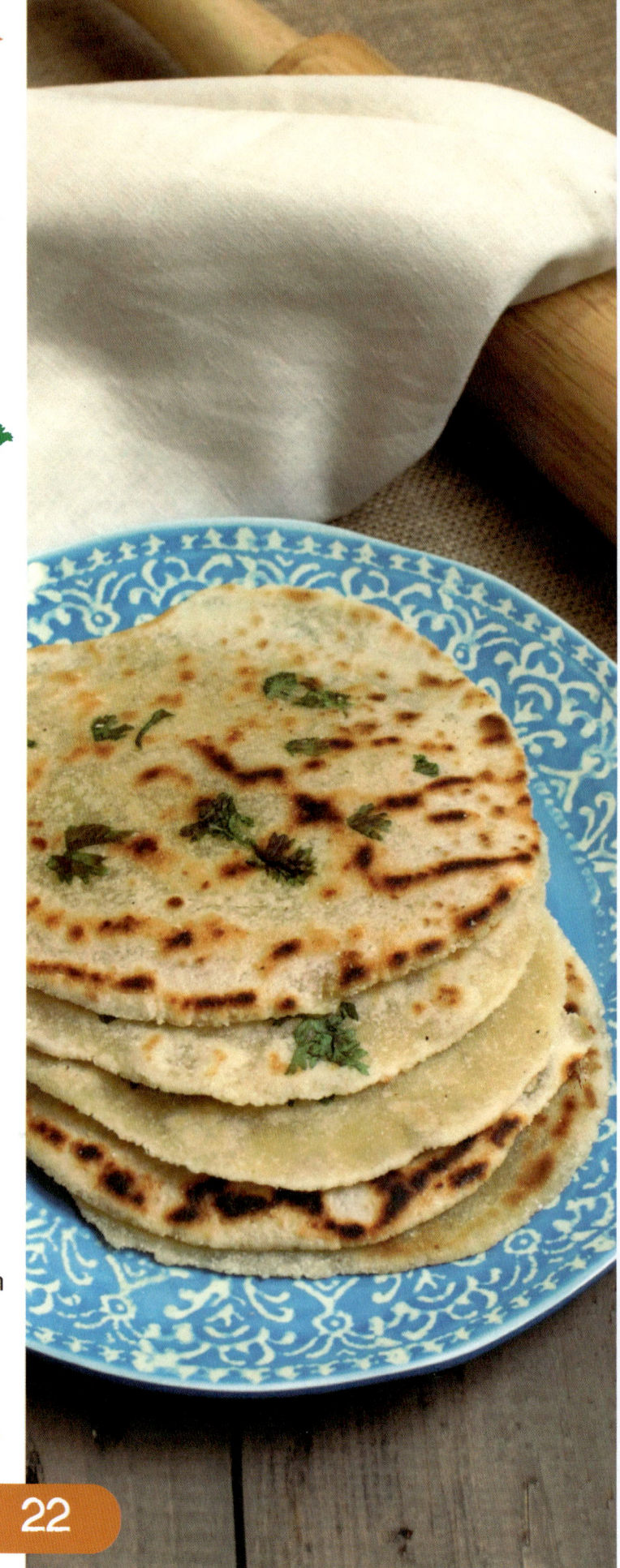

Ingredients:
- 1 1/4 cup + 2 TBSP cassava flour
- 1 tsp sea salt
- 1 tsp garlic granules
- 1/2 cup coconut milk
- 1/4 cup olive oil
- 2 TBSP cilantro leaves
- up to 3 TBSP water

Method:
- combine dry ingredients in a mixing bowl
- stir in coconut milk and olive oil and mix well with a fork to form a dough, then knead by hand
- desired dough is smooth and not sticky and able to roll into balls
- if dough is dry, add water until desired dough consistency is met
- place dough ball in the fridge to set for 10- 15 minutes
- divide the dough into 6 evenly sized balls
- use about 1/2 tsp cassava flour to dust each ball of dough before rolling
- roll each ball between 2 pieces of parchment paper to about 5-6 inch diameter
- press a few cilantro leaves into each roti
- heat a griddle pan or skillet over medium heat and drizzle with olive oil
- place roti on skillet and cook for 2-3 minutes on side one (until roti puffs up a bit)
- flip and cook another 1-2 minutes
- store in an airtight container in the fridge for a few days
- right before serving, microwave for 10 seconds in damp paper towel for soft and flexible roti

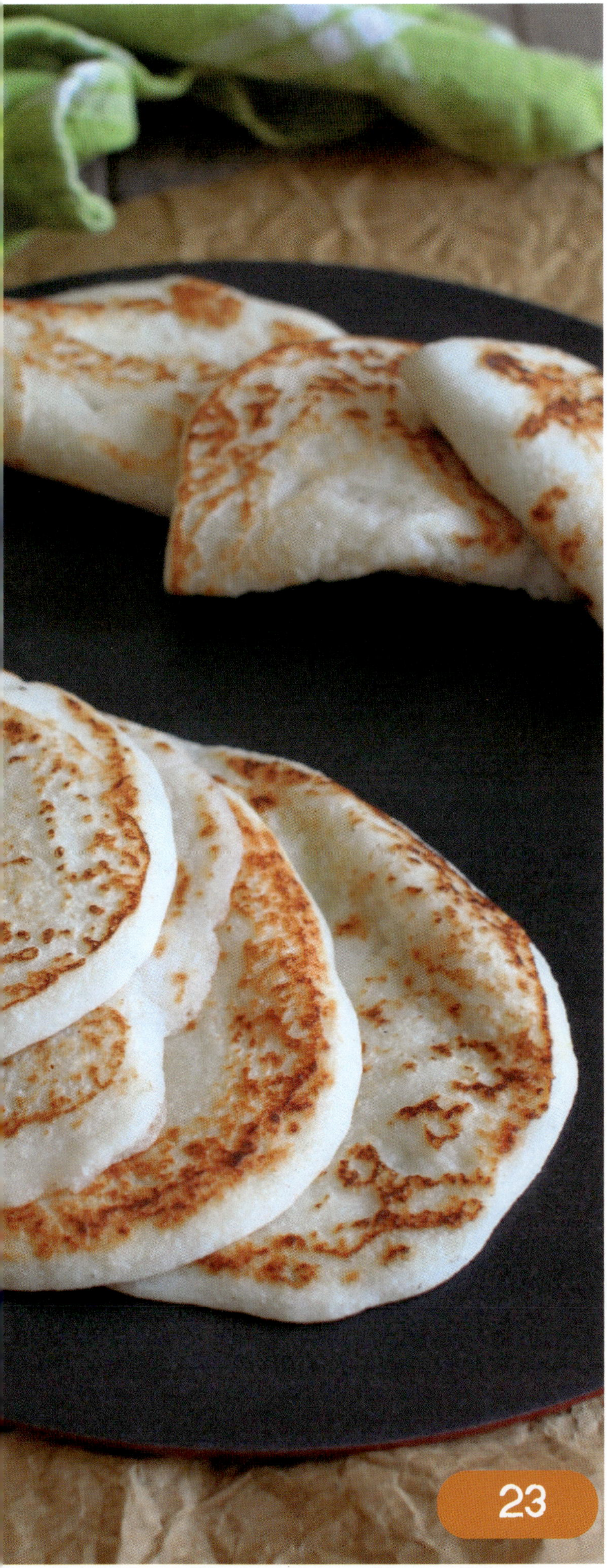

AIP Chapatis

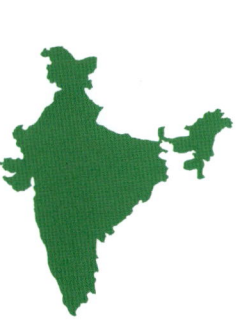

Ingredients:
- 1 TBSP coconut flour
- 2 TBSP arrowroot starch
  (or tapioca starch)
- 1/4 cup coconut milk
  (full fat)
- pinch of sea salt
- 1/2 TBSP coconut oil

Method:
- mix coconut flour, arrowroot starch, coconut milk and salt in a small bowl until well combined
- *(you may need to add a tsp of water if coconut milk is thick or less milk if your brand is very thin - you want pancake batter consistency)*
- heat coconut oil in a skillet over a low to medium heat.... NOTE - a non-stick pan is helpful for this recipe
- spoon the batter into the pan and use the back of the spoon to spread it around the pan
- cook for about 3 minutes on the first side. It should get bubbly like a pancake and the edges should start to brown.
- watch it carefully. You want it to cook slowly, so you may need to turn the heat down.
- carefully flip and cook the other side for 2 minutes
- drain on paper towels before eating

To make more than 1, simply multiply by the number of chapatis you want to make.

Stores well in the fridge a couple of days. Just reheat on paper towel in the microwave for 10 seconds.

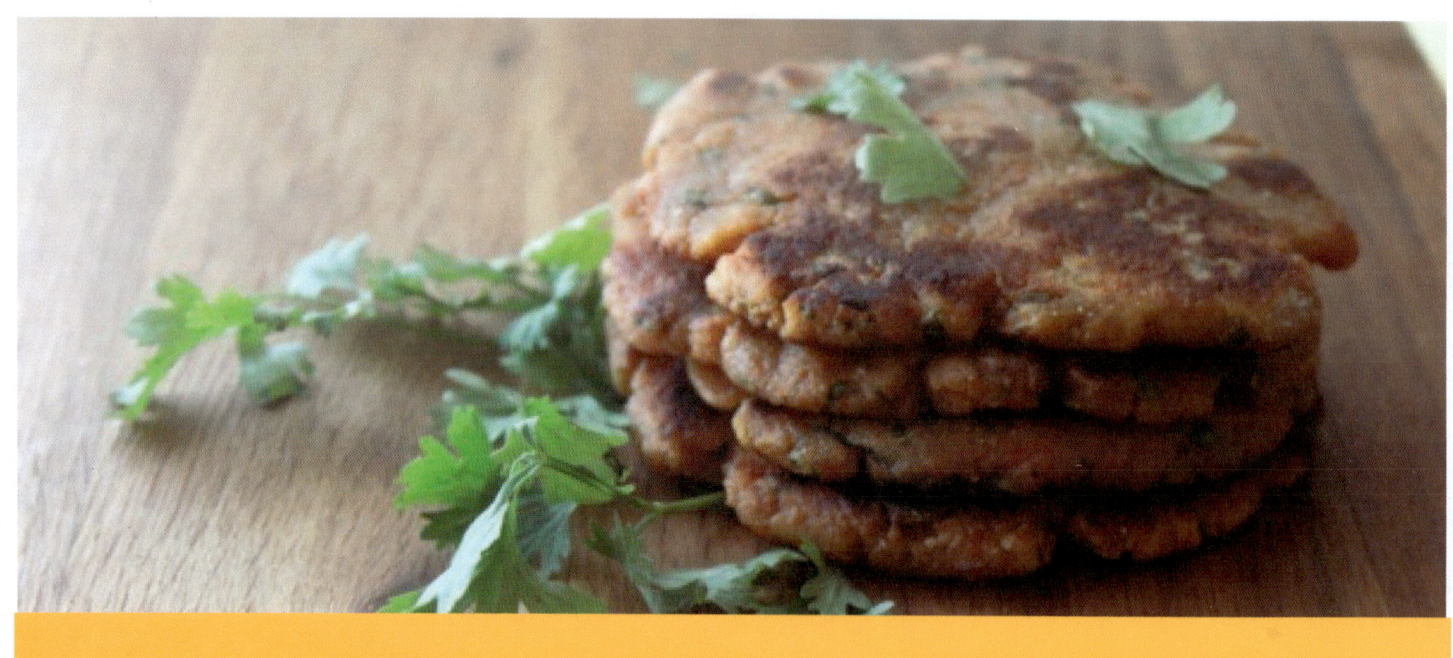

Sweet Potato Paratha

Serves: 3 · Time: 25 minutes

Ingredients:

- 1/3 cup mashed sweet potato - *just bake a sweet potato and scoop out the flesh*
- 1/2 cup cassava flour + 1 TBSP
- 1/2 tsp pink himalayan salt
- 1/2 tsp amchur (dried mango- optional)
- 1 TBSP chopped parsley
- 1 tsp coconut oil (liquid)
- 2 TBSP water
- oil for frying

Method:

- mix sweet potato, salt, amchur (if using) & parsley
- add in 1/2 cup cassava flour, and using a fork mix into the sweet potato mixture
- add in the coconut oil and mix to form a sand like consistency
- add 2 TBSP water (1 TBSP at a time), mixing until the dough pulls away from the bowl and forms a ball
- the dough should be wet - sprinkle in the remaining 1 TBSP cassava flour and begin to mix it together with your hands - at this point you might need to add 1/2-1 TBSP more flour if the dough still feels too wet
- divide into 3 pieces
- place a piece of parchment paper on the counter, dust a piece of the dough with cassava flour, cover with another piece of parchment paper and roll out to about 5 inches
- heat a small amount of coconut oil in a skillet over medium heat
- fry parathas for about 3 minutes on each side until they begin to brown around the edges

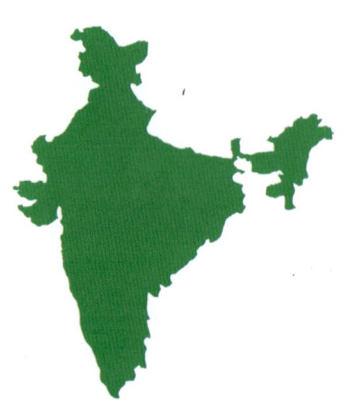

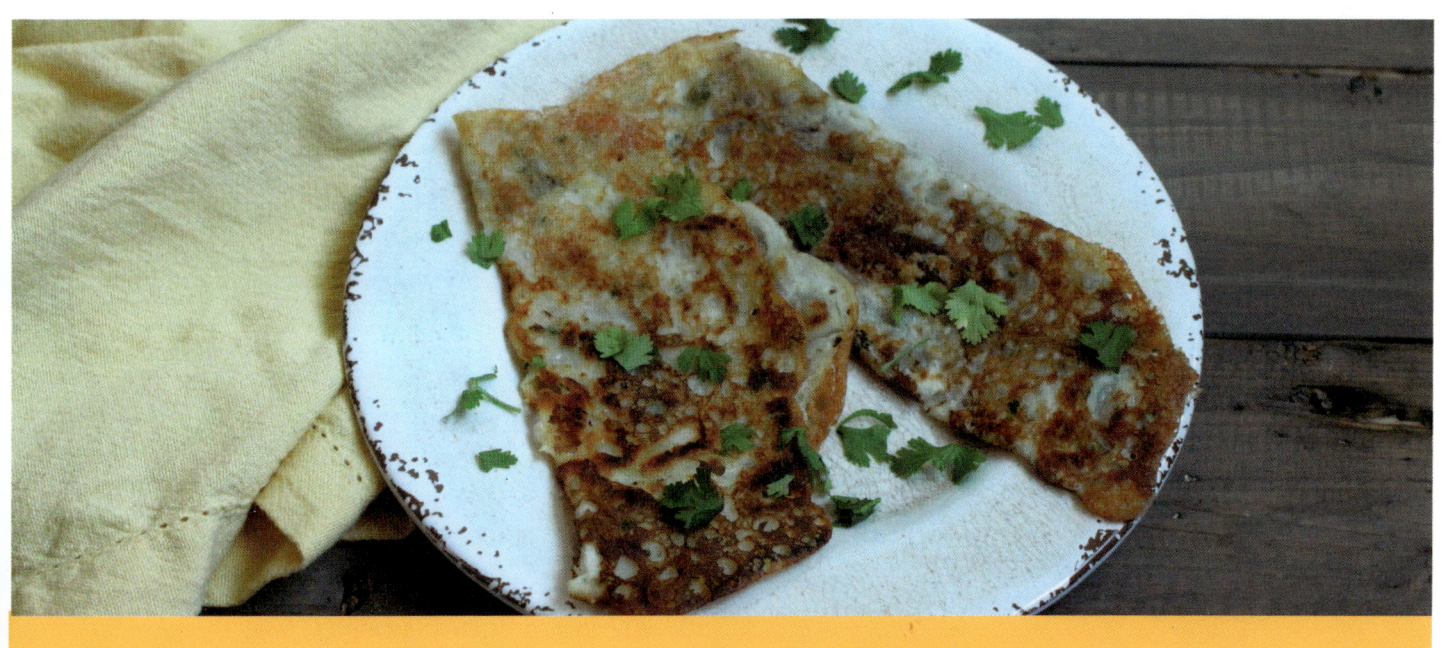

Onion Dosa

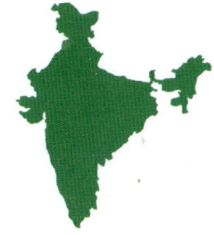

Makes: 6   Time: 50 minutes

Ingredients:

- 1/2 cup cassava flour
- 1/4 cup coconut flour
- 1/4 cup finely diced onion
- 2 TBSP chopped fresh cilantro
- 3/4 tsp pink himalayan salt
- 1 tsp dried ginger
- 2 cups water
- olive oil for frying

For a traditional taste, turn the dosa into 'masala dosa' by filling it with 'spicy alu makha' (pg. 74) and enjoy eating it with your hands.

Method:

- mix all ingredients to form a thin batter and set to the side for 15 minutes
- heat a skillet or griddle over medium heat
- drizzle with a bit of olive oil
- using a ladle pour about 1/2 cup batter onto the griddle in a circular motion starting with the outside of the dosa (about a 7 inch circle) and working toward the middle... the goal is thin and lacy, but if the holes are large add a bit more batter to fill the gaps
- turn heat to low and drizzle a bit of olive oil (1/2 tsp) over the top and around the edges, turning the pan to get oil around the edges
- allow to cook for 3 minutes
- be patient and don't try to flip too soon, but wait for it brown around the edges
- flip over and allow to cook an additional 2-3 minutes
- flip again and fold in half then cook about 1 minute on each side
- eat with coconut chutney (pg. 31) for a snack or easy breakfast.
- best served hot, but once cooled can be kept in the fridge

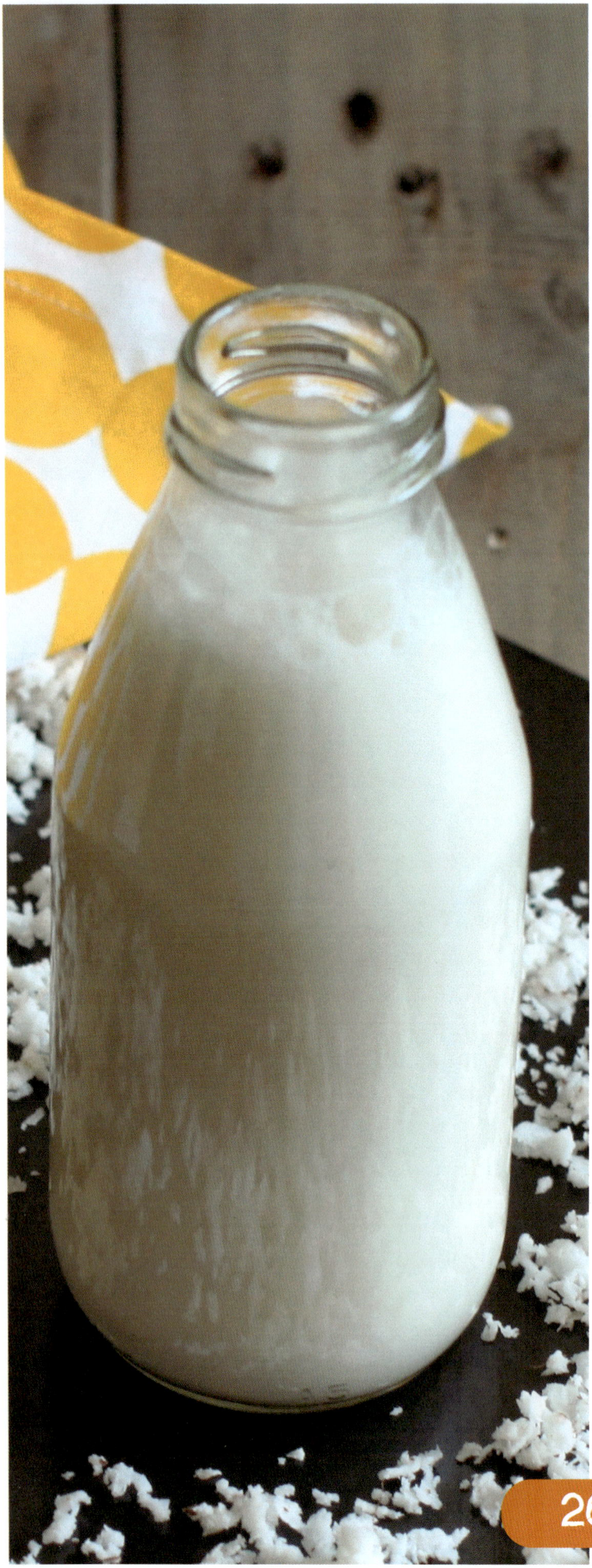

Coconut Milk

Makes: 2 cups   Time: 10 minutes

Ingredients:
- 1 cup of fresh grated coconut or dried shredded coconut
- 2 cups of hot (boiling) water - 2 1/2 cups if using dried coconut

Method:
- place coconut in a blender jar
- pour hot water over coconut
- allow to sit for 2-3 minutes
- blend until smooth
- if using for curry - leave as is
- if using for a drink or ice cream - strain through a fine sieve (or cheesecloth)
- store in the fridge for up to a week
- milk will separate, so shake well or blend again before using.

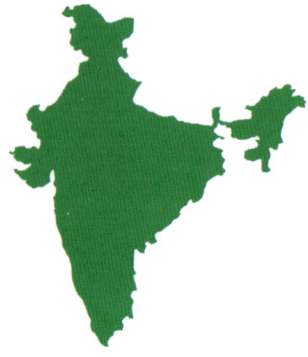

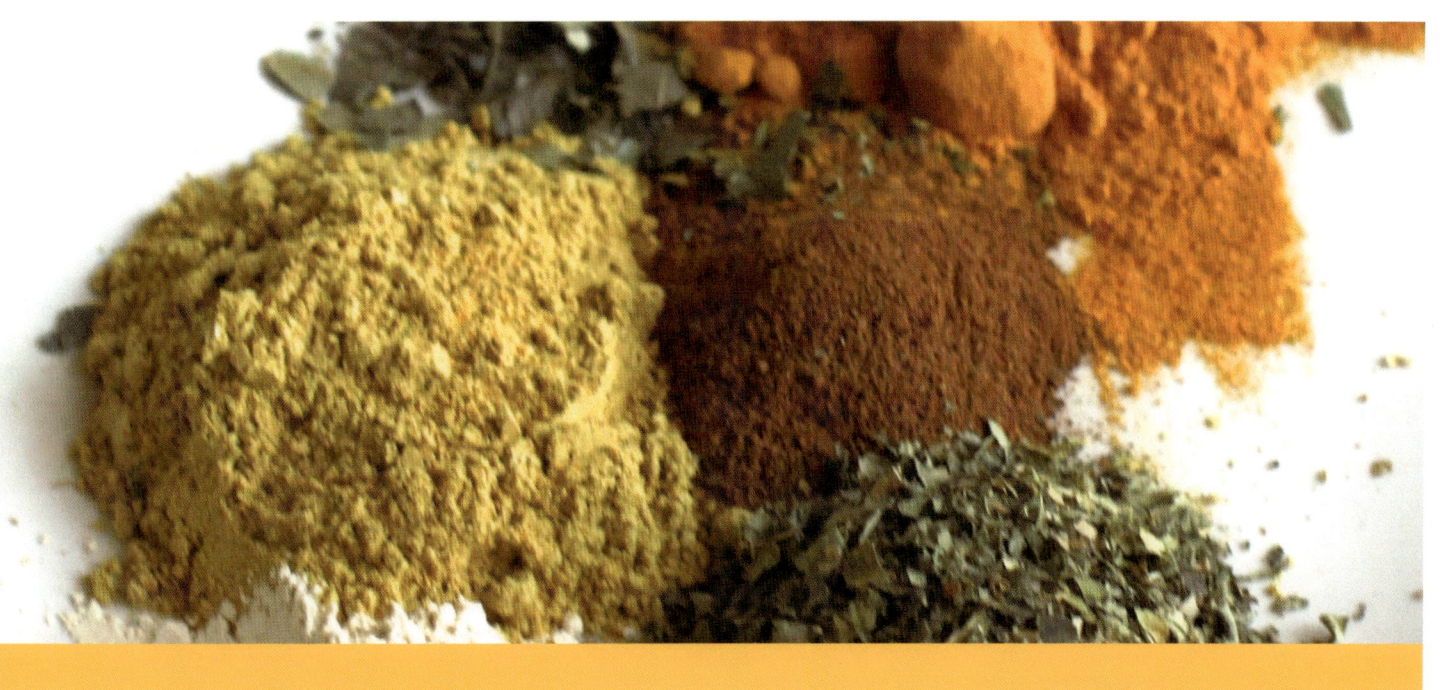

AIP/Paleo Curry Powder

<u>Time</u>: 5 minutes

Ingredients:
- 2 Tbsp powdered ginger
- 1 Tbsp powdered garlic
- 2 Tbsp powdered turmeric
- 2 tsp ground cinnamon
- 1/2 tsp ground cloves
- 1/2 tsp ground mace
- 2 Tbsp dried cilantro/ coriander leaves
- 1 tsp fenugreek leaves
- 1 tsp crushed curry leaves

Make a batch of this and store in an airtight jar. Use it anytime you see garam masala or curry powder listed in a recipe.

Method:
- Mix all ingredients well and store in a glass jar for future use.
- If the cilantro, curry & fenugreek are large leaves, you may way to crush them in a mortar & pestle or a spice grinder.

<u>Reintroduction Note</u>:
*If you've reintroduced seed based spices (stage one reintroduction), you may want to add one or more of the following for a more **'traditional'** taste.*

- 1 Tbsp ground cumin
- 1 Tbsp ground coriander seeds
- 1/2 tsp dry mustard or 1 tsp mustard seeds
- 1 tsp black pepper

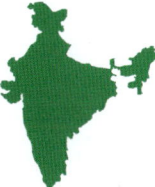

Coconut Turmeric Rice

Serves: 4   Time: 20 minutes

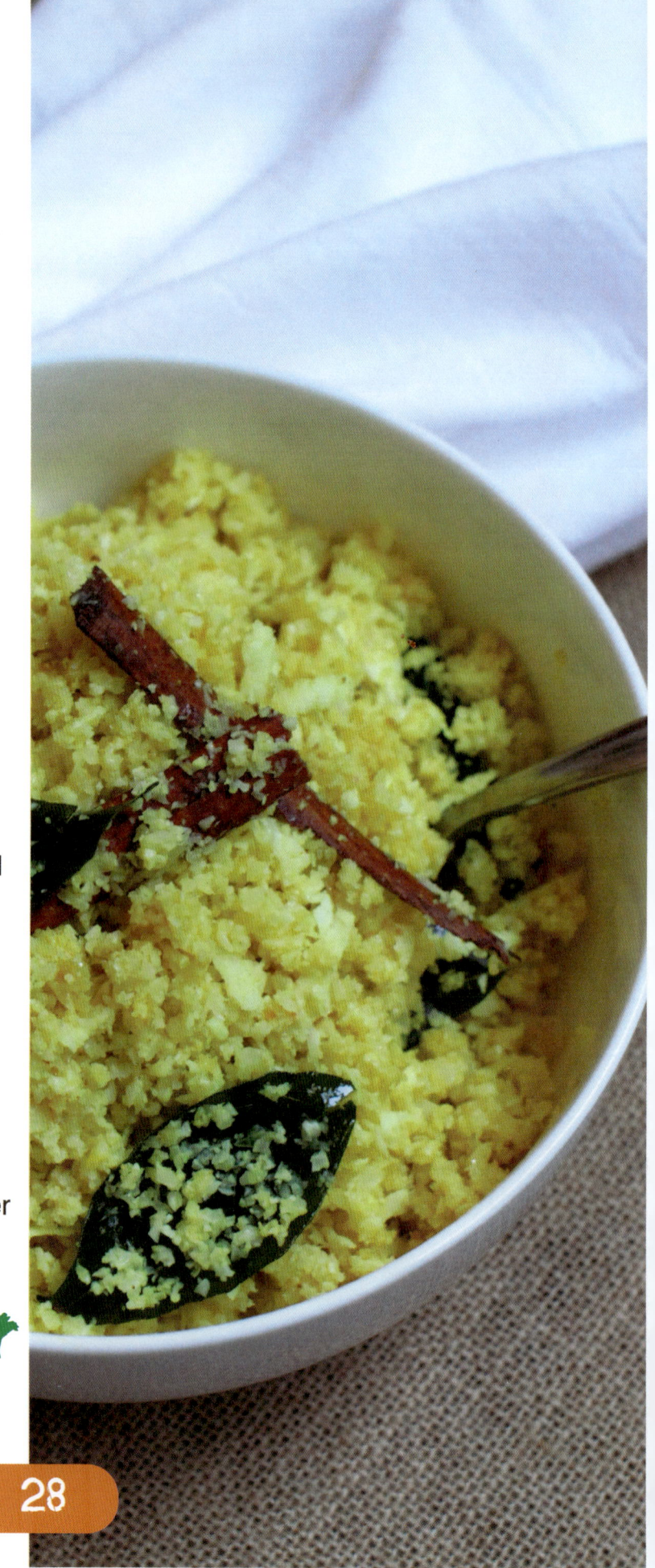

Ingredients:
- small head of cauliflower
- 2 TBSP coconut oil
- 1/2 red onion
- 1/2 tsp turmeric
- 1/2 tsp ginger powder
- 8 cloves
- 1/2 tsp pink himalayan salt
- 6 curry leaves
- 1 cinnamon stick -broken in half
- 1/4 cup fresh grated coconut
- 1/4 cup water

Method:
- cut cauliflower into florets and use a food processor or box grater to grate into 'rice' like pieces
- finely dice an onion
- heat coconut oil in a large skillet over medium heat
- add onion, curry leaves, cinnamon sticks and all spices to hot oil - stir fry until spices are fragrant
- add grated cauliflower, coconut and water and stir in well
- reduce heat to low and cook 6-8 minutes until water cooks off and cauliflower is fluffy like rice

28

TIP: many Indian dishes begin with a combination of onion, garlic and ginger. If you plan on doing a lot of Indian cooking in the next couple of days, consider making a paste of the three with a pinch of salt in your mortar and pestle or food processor and storing it in the fridge.

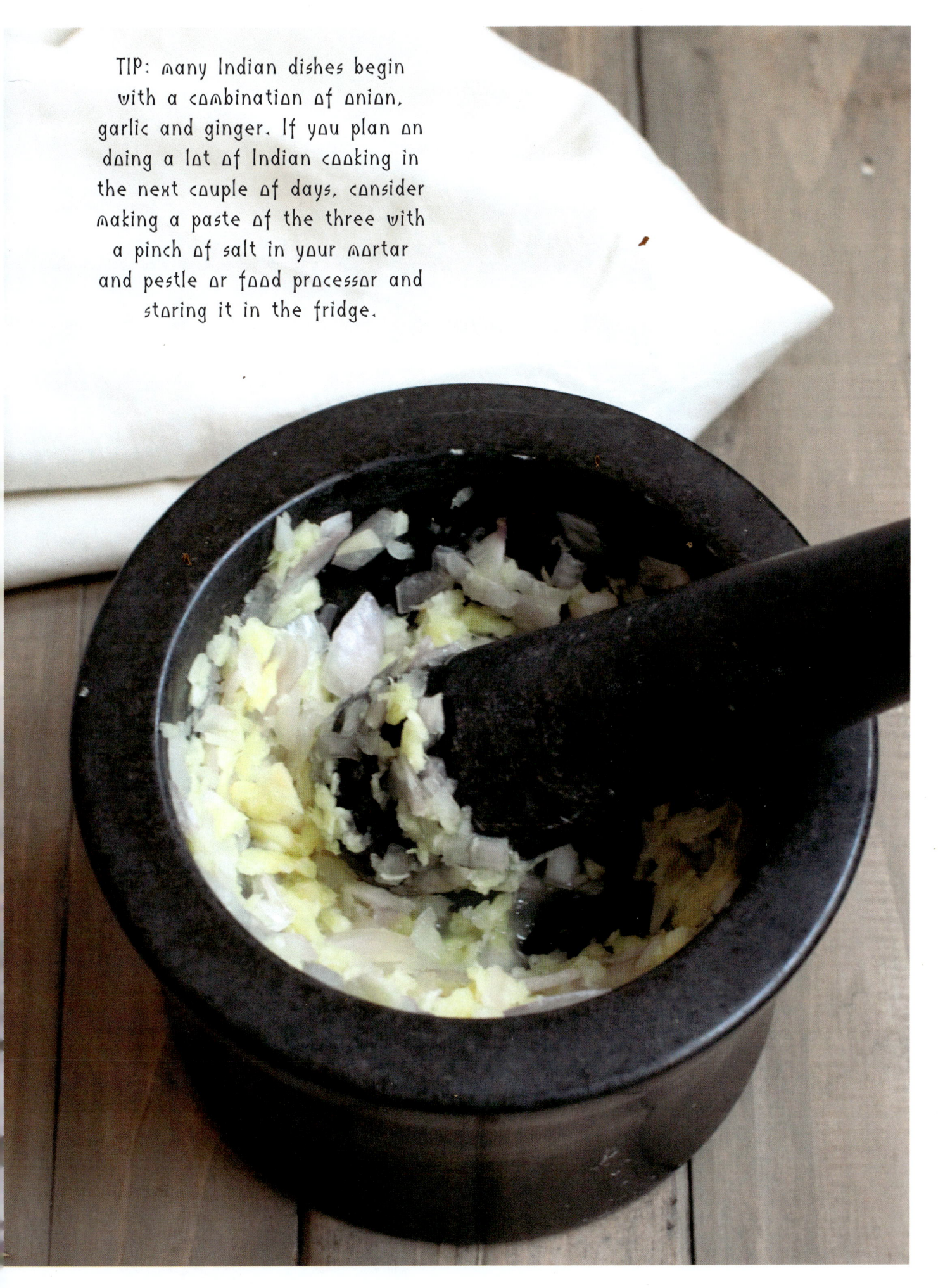

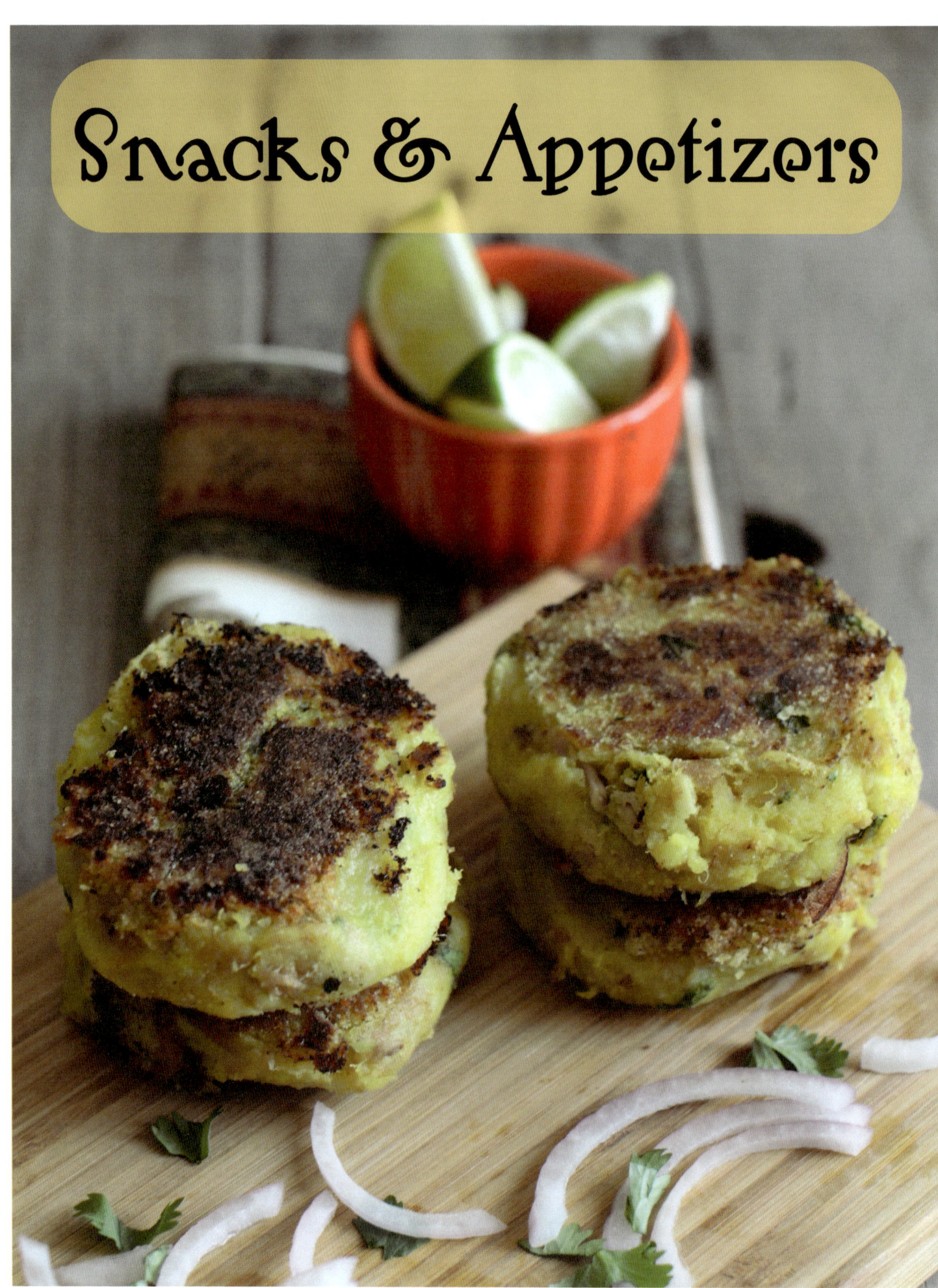

Snacks & Appetizers

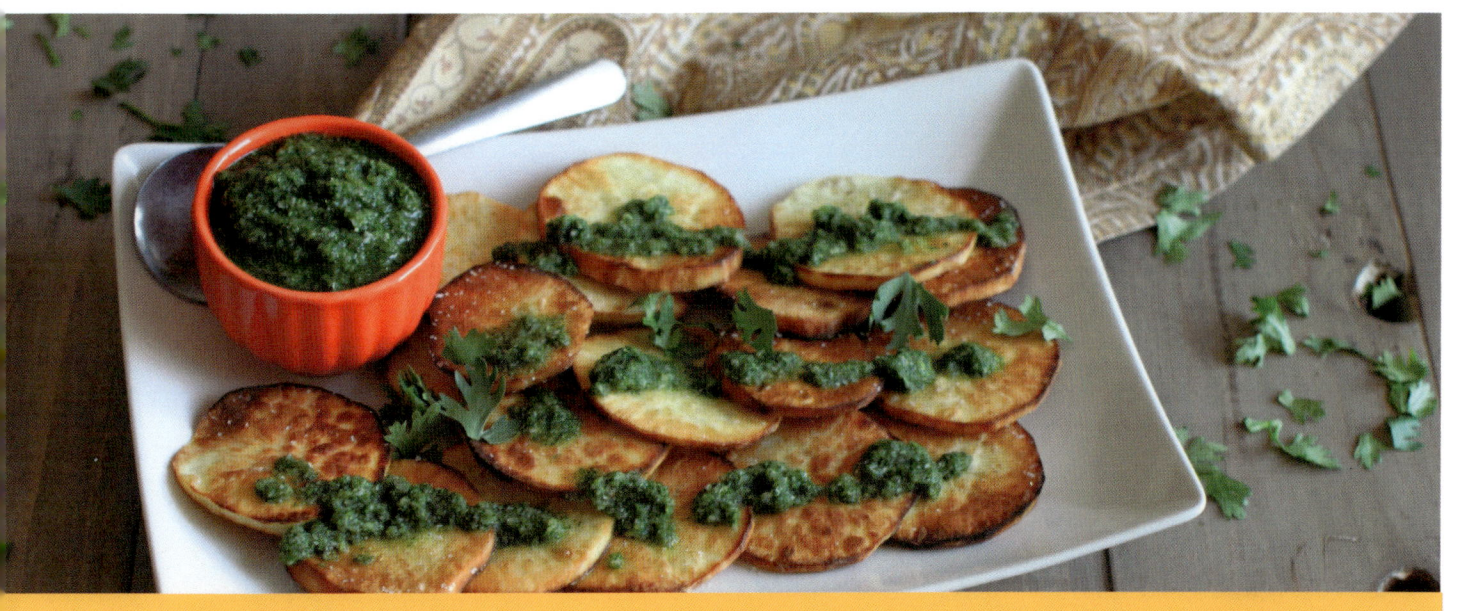

Coriander Chutney

Serves: 6   Time: 5 minutes

Ingredients:
- 1 inch piece of ginger
- 4- 5 cloves of garlic
- 1/2 of a medium red onion
- 3 handfuls of cilantro/ coriander leaves
- 1/2 tsp pink himalayan salt
- juice of 1 lime
- 1/2 TBSP apple cider vinegar
- 2 TBSP water

Having several chutneys available can completely change the taste of a dish and allows your family to personalize based on their tastes.

Method:
- peel and rough chop the ginger and garlic
- rough chop the onion
- place all ingredients in a food processor and process until you achieve a smooth consistency
- serve as a topping for curry, use as a marinade for 'coriander prawn skewers' (pg. 68), dip pieces of roti (pg. 22), or sprinkle over 'cassava thoran' (pg. 76).

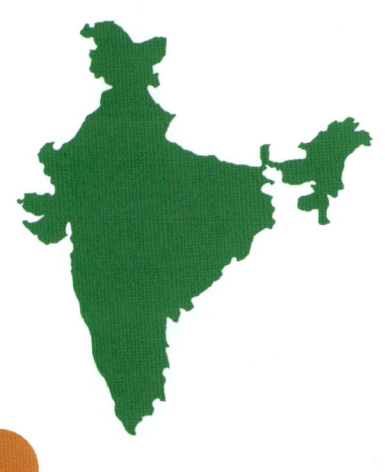

Mango Ginger Chutney

Serves: 6   Time: 45 minutes

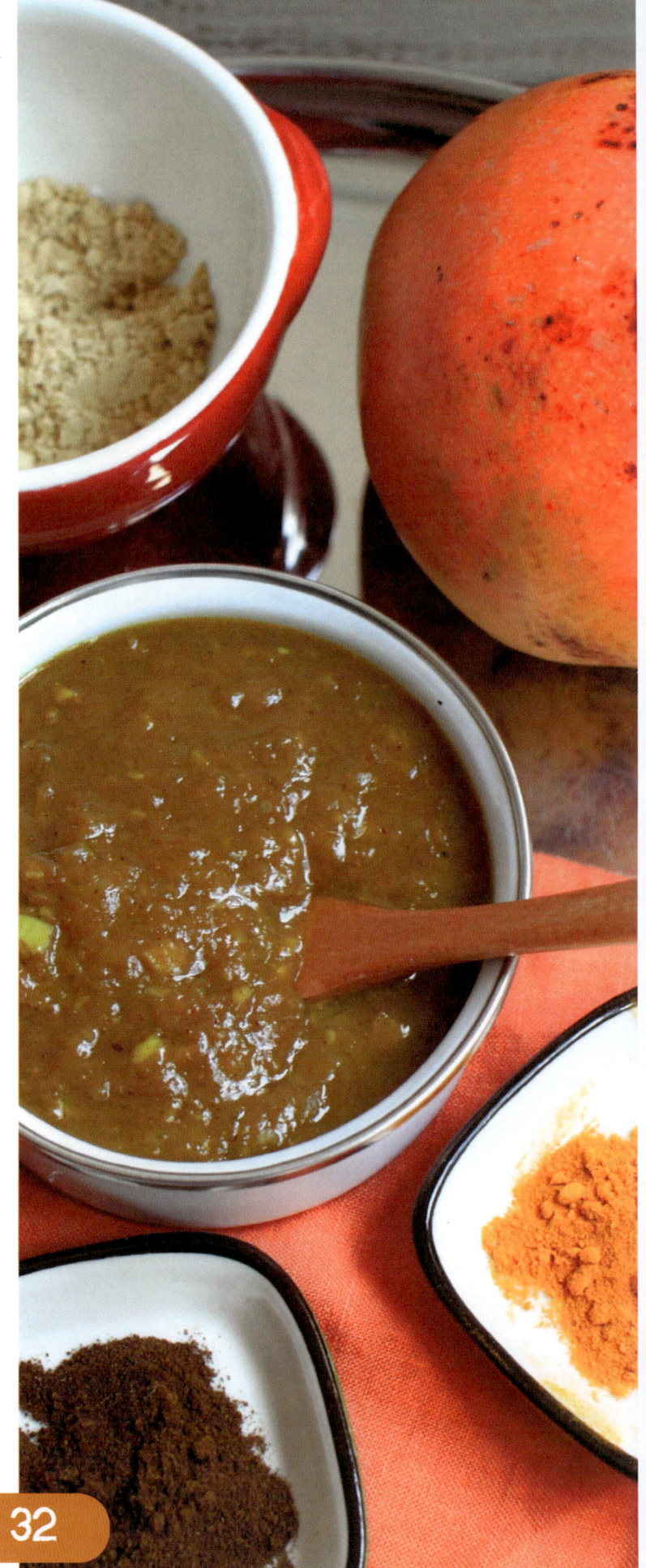

Ingredients:
- 2 TBSP Coconut oil
- 1/2 red onion
- 2 cloves garlic
- 2 inch piece of ginger
- 1/2 tsp turmeric
- 1 tsp ginger powder
- 1/4 tsp cinnamon
- 1/4 tsp cloves
- 1 tsp pink himalayan salt
- 1 large mango
- 2 TBSP coconut sugar ✳ 1 TBSP
- 1/4 cup apple cider vinegar
- 1/4 cup water

Method:
- place 1/2 onion, 2 cloves garlic and fresh ginger in a food processor and pulse until finely chopped
- peel and chop mango into small pieces
- heat coconut oil in a saucepan over medium heat
- add onion, garlic ginger mixture and sauté for 1-2 minutes
- add spices and continue cooking (while stirring) until fragrant and onions are soft
- add mango, coconut sugar, apple cider vinegar and water to the saucepan and reduce heat to low
- allow to simmer for 30 minutes or until water has cooked off and chutney thickens.

Reintroduction Note:

If you can eat seed spices, add 1/2 tsp cumin seeds and 1/2 tsp coriander seeds with the onion, garlic and ginger.

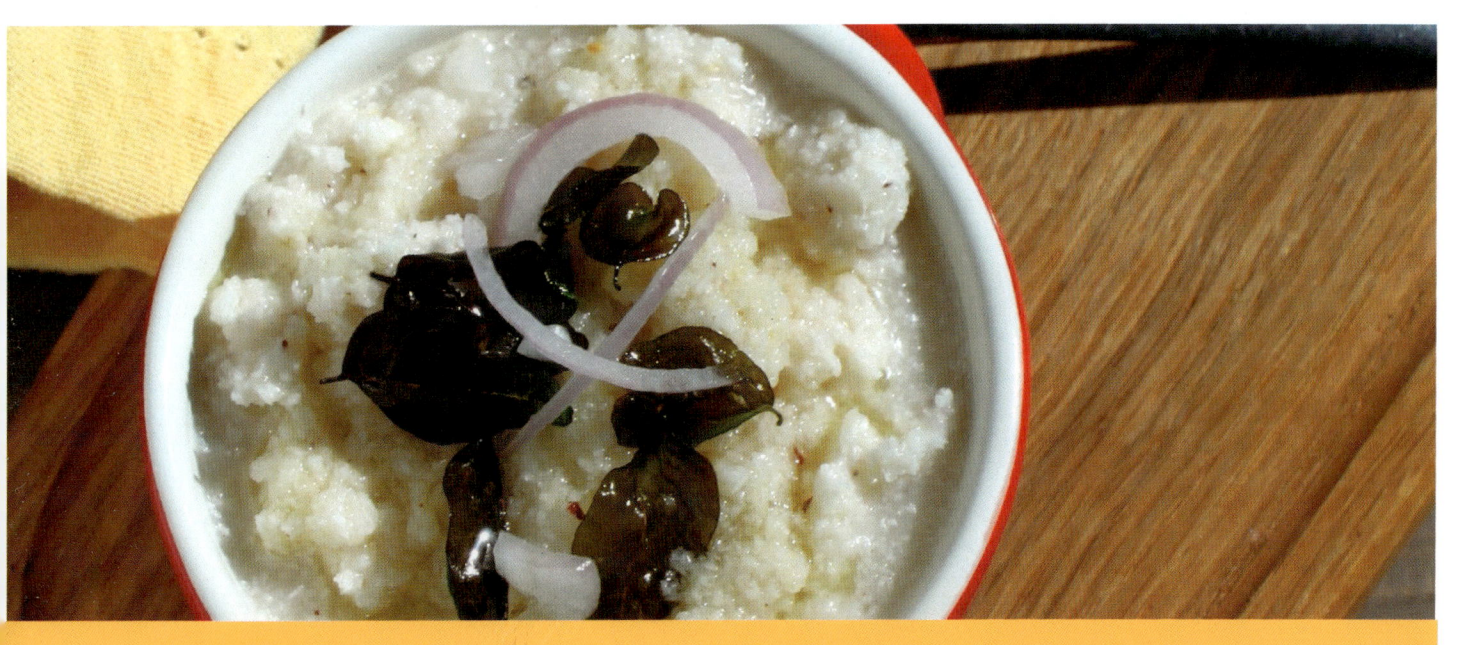

Coconut Chutney

Serves: 6   Time: 5 minutes

Ingredients:
- 1/2 cup fresh grated coconut
- 1 small (or 1/2 medium) red onion
- 1/2 tsp ginger powder
- 1/2 tsp pink salt
- 1/2 tsp garlic powder
- 1/4 cup water
- 8-10 curry leaves
- 1/2 TBSP olive oil

Method:
- rough chop the onion
- place coconut, onion, ginger, garlic, salt & water in a food processor and blend until onion is finely chopped and all ingredients are well combined
- transfer coconut mixture to a small bowl
- heat olive oil in a small skillet over a low heat
- once hot, add curry leaves to the oil and sauté until curry leaves are crisp
- spoon the curry leaves and olive oil over the chutney
- serve alongside your favorite curry or enjoy with an onion dosa (pg. 25) or roti (pg. 22) for a quick breakfast

Reintroduction Note:
If you can eat seed spices, temper 1/2 tsp mustard seeds with the curry leaves.

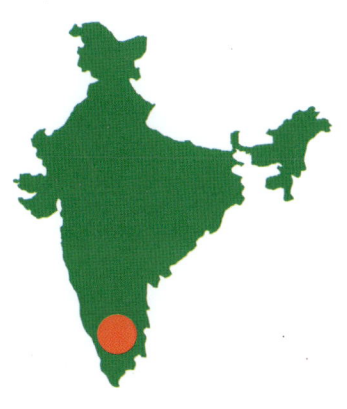

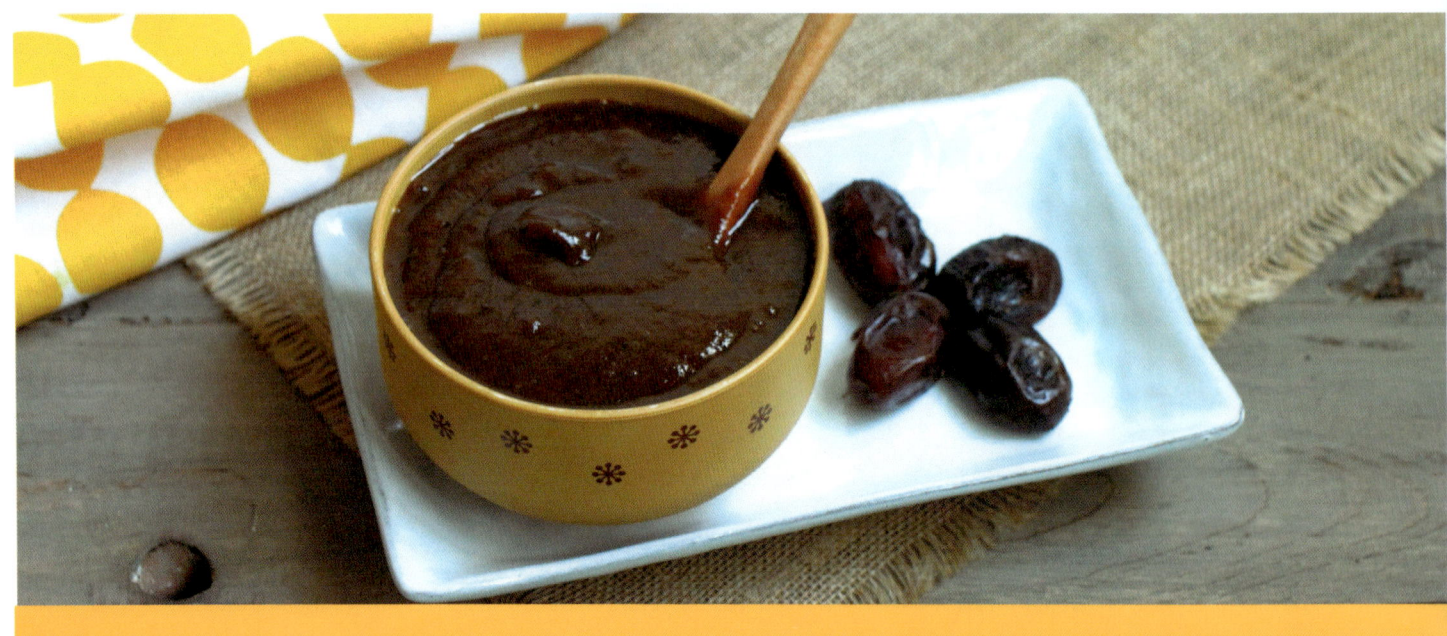

Date Tamarind Chutney

Makes: 1 cup   Time: 35 minutes

Ingredients:
- 1/4 cup of tamarind pulp
- 3/4 cup warm water
- 1/2 cup of dates - seeds removed
- 1 TBSP coconut sugar
- 1/4 tsp sea salt
- 1 tsp ginger powder
- 1/8 tsp mace
- 1/8 tsp cinnamon
- 1/4 tsp turmeric
- 1/4 tsp amchur powder
- 1.5 cups water

Method:
- soak tamarind pulp in warm water for 5 minutes - then use your fingers to remove the seeds and large fibrous pieces
- add deseeded dates to the tamarind water
- add remaining ingredients
- simmer on low for 25-30 minutes until liquid has reduced and dates and tamarind have broken down *(you want a BBQ sauce/ ketchup kind of consistency)*
- use an immersion blender to blend until smooth
- if fibrous bits of tamarind or date are still present, strain through a sieve
- keeps in the fridge for 2 weeks
- serve with samosas (pg. 43), bajis, fried sweet potatoes and other snacks. This chutney is perfect for chaat (pg. 45).

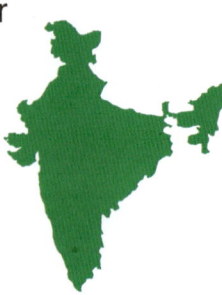

This chutney also makes a fantastic BBQ sauce for the days you want an non-Indian dinner... it's great on burgers and meatloaf

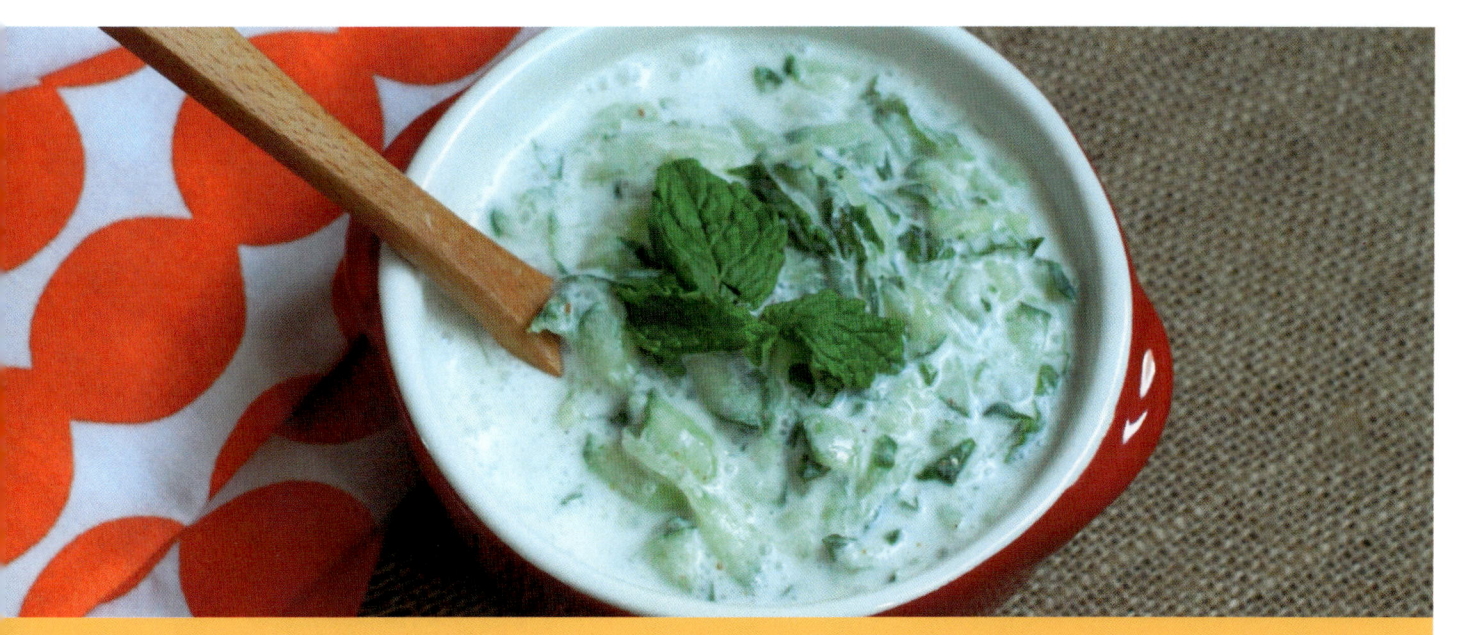

Cucumber Mint Raita

Makes: 1 cup   Time: 15 minutes

Ingredients:
- 2 medium cucumbers
- 2 TBSP chopped mint leaves
- 1/2 cup coconut milk
- 1/8 tsp mace
- 1/4 tsp ginger
- 1 tsp lemon juice
- 1/4 tsp pink himalayan salt

Method:
- grate cucumbers
- squeeze as much water out of the cucumber as you can and place in a dry bowl
- finely chop the mint leaves
- mix all ingredients except salt
- add salt right before serving
- use as a topping for biryani or fried king fish

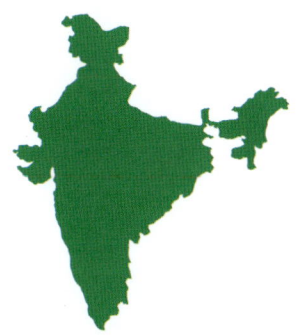

This raita is also great for with spiced lamb kebabs (pg. 53) and has a great cooling effect when served with curries.

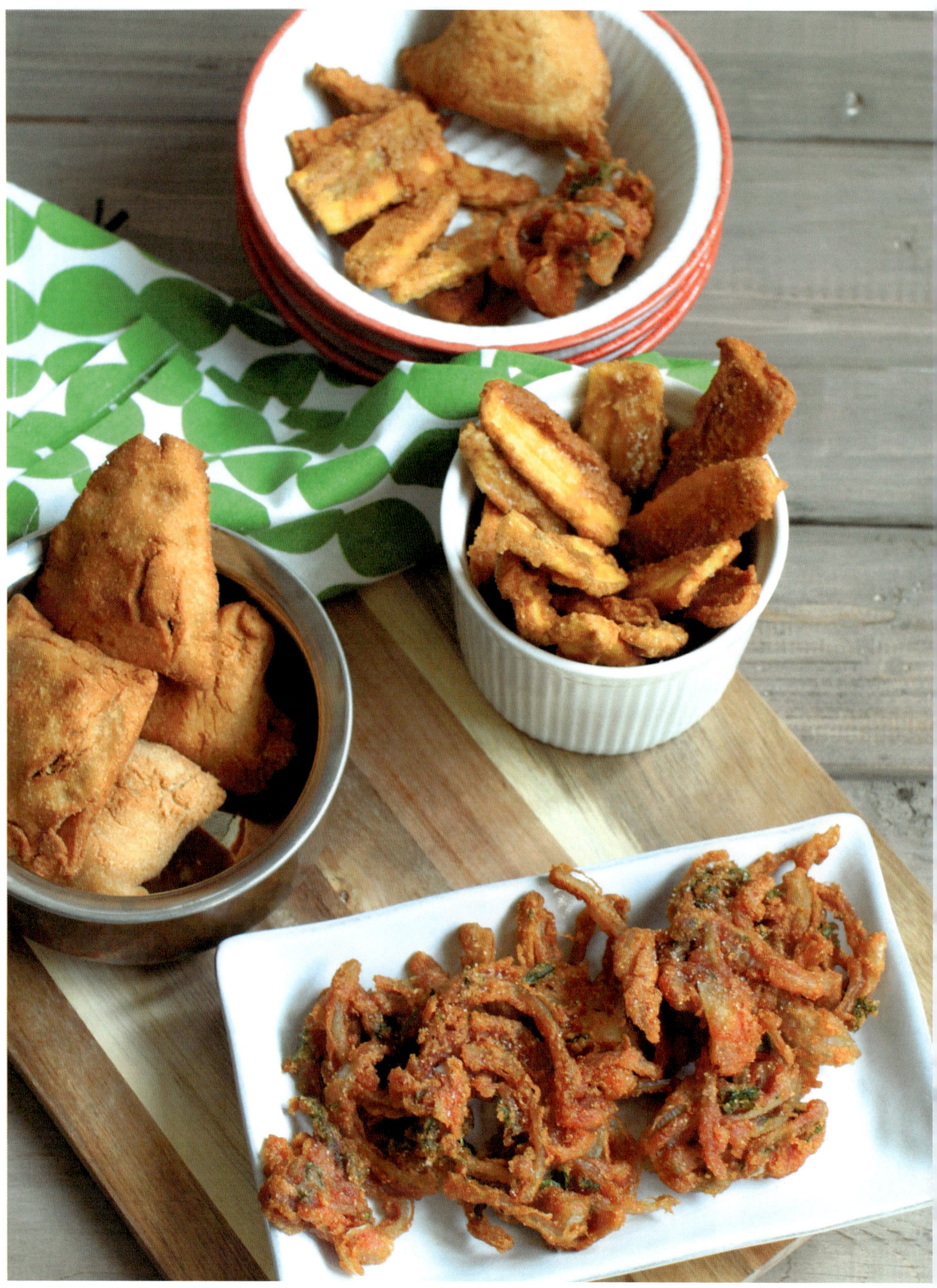

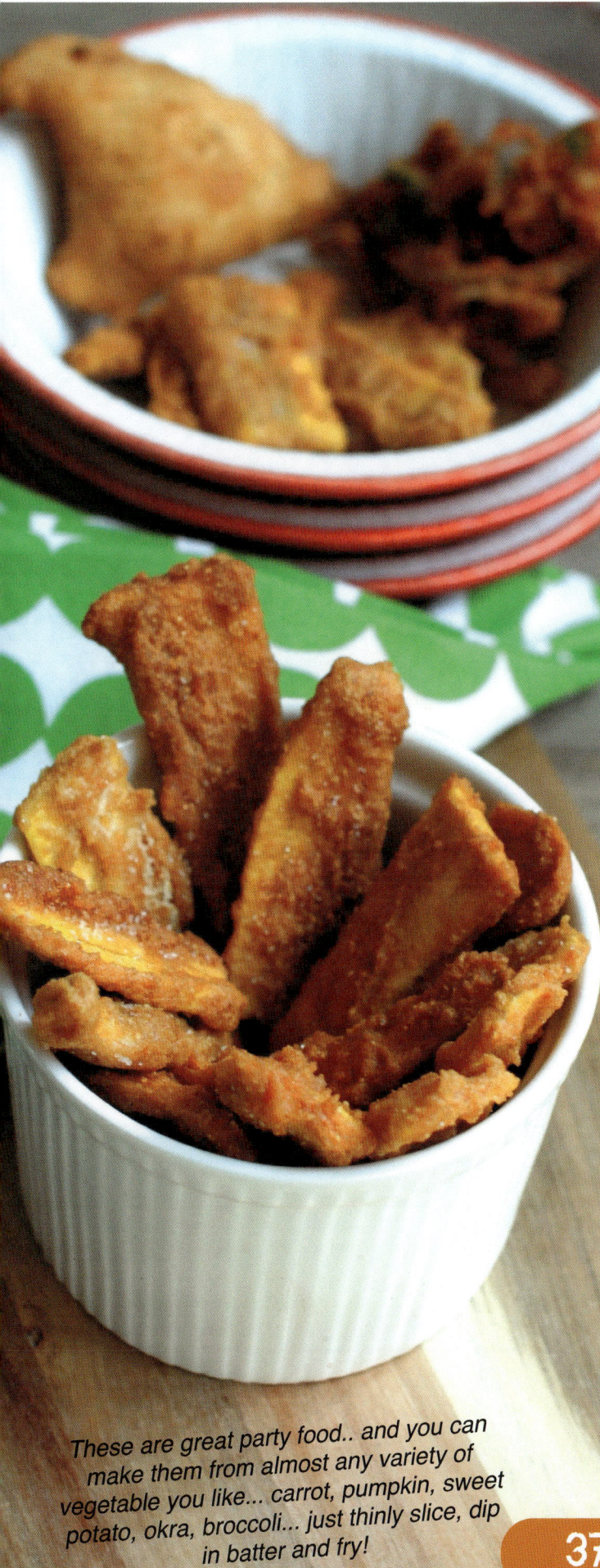

Plantain Bajjis

Serves: 3-4   Time: 25 minutes

Ingredients:

- 1 large green plantain
- 1/2 cup cassava flour
- 1/8 tsp turmeric
- 1/4 tsp dried ginger
- 1/4 tsp garlic powder
- 1/4 tsp baking soda
- 1/4 tsp sea salt
- 6 TBSP water
- coconut oil to deep fry

Method:

- heat coconut oil in a saucepan over medium heat - needs to be about 3 inches deep
- peel plantains and cut into 3 inch pieces and thinly slice - lengthwise (as thin as you can)
- mix remaining ingredients (except oil) in a medium sized bowl. You're goal is a batter consistency
- add the sliced plantains to the bowl and mix well to coat all of the plantain slices with the batter
- check oil - drop a small piece of plantain into the oil - it should bubble all around and rise to the top of the oil
- drop 6-7 pieces of plantains into the oil at a time being sure not to crowd them
- flip them over a few times with a slotted spoon while they fry over low to medium heat for about 4 minutes
- remove to a paper towel lined plate to cool
- serve with chutney of choice - mango is my favorite

These are great party food.. and you can make them from almost any variety of vegetable you like... carrot, pumpkin, sweet potato, okra, broccoli... just thinly slice, dip in batter and fry!

Kachumber Salad

Serves: 4-6   Time: 10 minutes

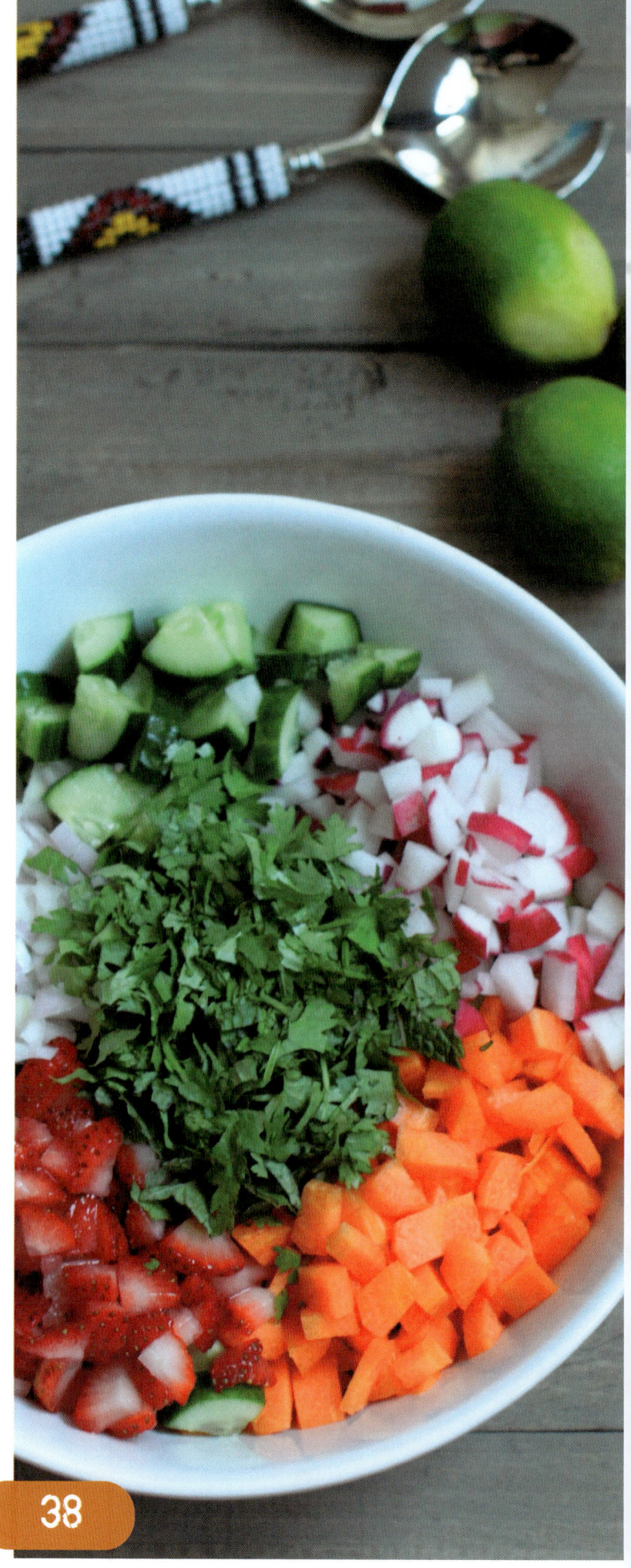

Ingredients:
• 4 medium cucumbers
• 1 medium carrot
• 5 red radishes
• 1 medium red onion
• 6-8 strawberries
• 12 mint leaves
• 1/4 cup cilantro leaves
• Juice of 2 limes
• 1/2 tsp ginger powder
• 1/4 tsp pink himalayan salt

Method:
• wash and chop all the vegetables into a small dice size
• finely shred the mint and cilantro leaves
• combine the lime juice, ginger and salt in a small bowl and stir well to combine
• pour the dressing over the salad and toss well to combine

Reintroduction Note:
If you can handle tomatoes, use cherry tomatoes instead of strawberries as they are more traditional in this salad.

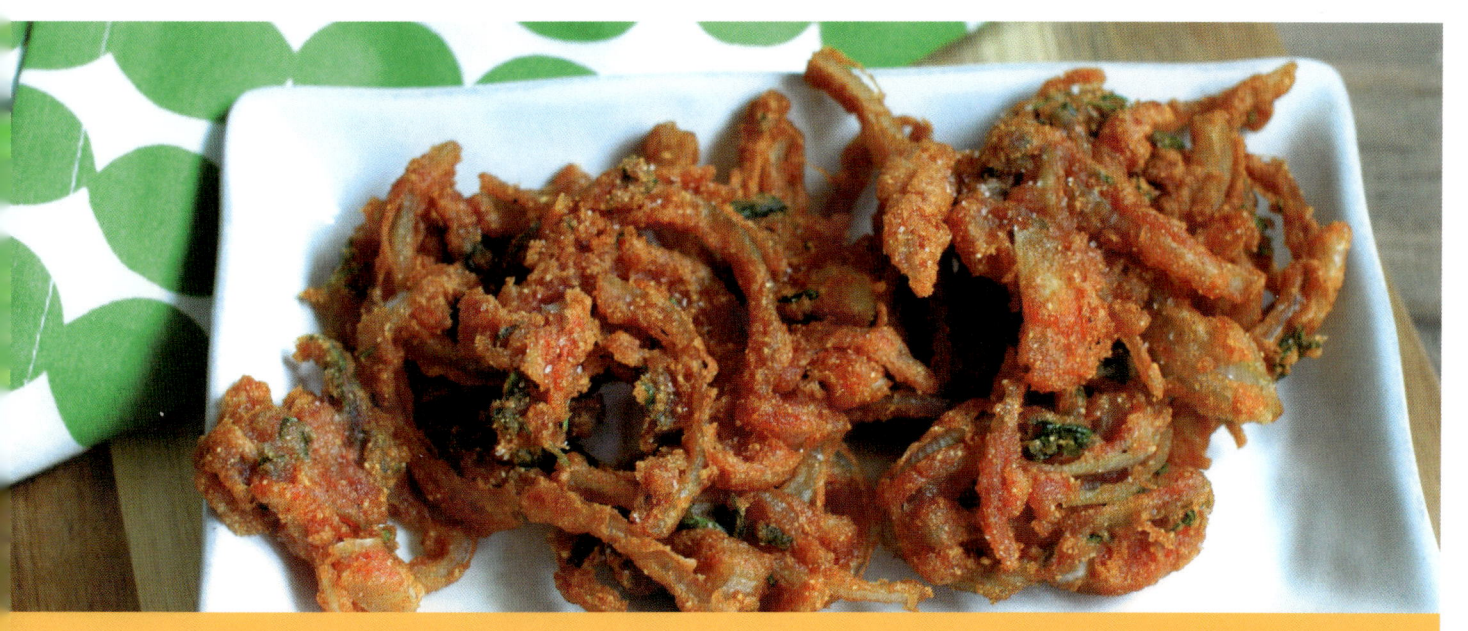

Onion Bajjis

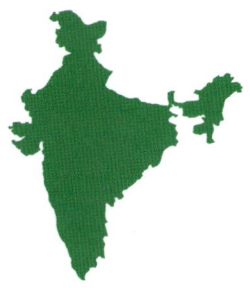

Serves: 4-6   Time: 30 minutes

Ingredients:
- 1 large white or red onion
- 1/3 cup cassava flour
- 1/2 tsp pink himalayan salt
- 1/4 tsp baking soda
- 1/2 tsp dried ginger
- 1/4 tsp turmeric
- 1 TBSP fresh cilantro/ coriander leaves
- 3-4 TBSP water
- coconut oil for deep frying (about 2 inches deep in the pan)

Consider serving along with plantain bajis and fish cutlets the next time you need some heavy appetizers at a game or party.

Method:
- cut onion in half and then slice thinly into 1/2 moon shapes and divide all of the onion pieces
- heat coconut oil in a saucepan over medium heat - about 2-3 inches deep
- mix remaining ingredients (except oil) in a medium sized bowl. You're goal is a thick batter
- add the onions to the bowl and mix well to coat all of the onion slices with the batter
- check oil - drop a small piece of onion into the oil - it should bubble all around and rise to the top of the oil
- once oil is hot, take a spoonful of the onion batter mixture and drop into hot oil
- fry 2-3 bajjis at a time being careful not to crowd them
- bajjis fry for 3-4 minutes until golden brown
- remove to a paper towel lined plate to cool
- TIP: if onion pieces are coming apart, hold together with a spoon while they fry
- serve with coriander chutney (pg. 31)

Turmeric Sweet Potatoes

Serves: 4-6   Time: 25 minutes

Ingredients:
- 2 medium white flesh sweet potatoes
- 1/4 tsp turmeric
- 1/4 tsp pink himalayan salt
- 3-4 TBSP coconut oil

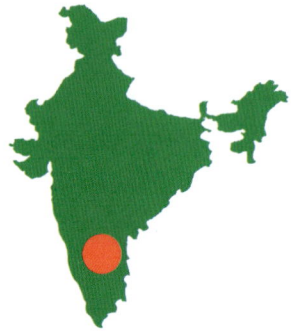

Method:
- thinly slice the sweet potatoes
- sprinkle turmeric and salt over the sweet potatoes and toss to combine
- heat coconut oil over medium heat in a large skillet
- fry sweet potatoes about 2 minutes on each side and remove to a paper towel lined plate to drain the oil
- sprinkle with more salt after cooking
- you'll need to cook the sweet potatoes in 2 or 3 batches
- serve with some Date & Tamarind Chutney and/or Coriander Chutney for a fun snack or side dish

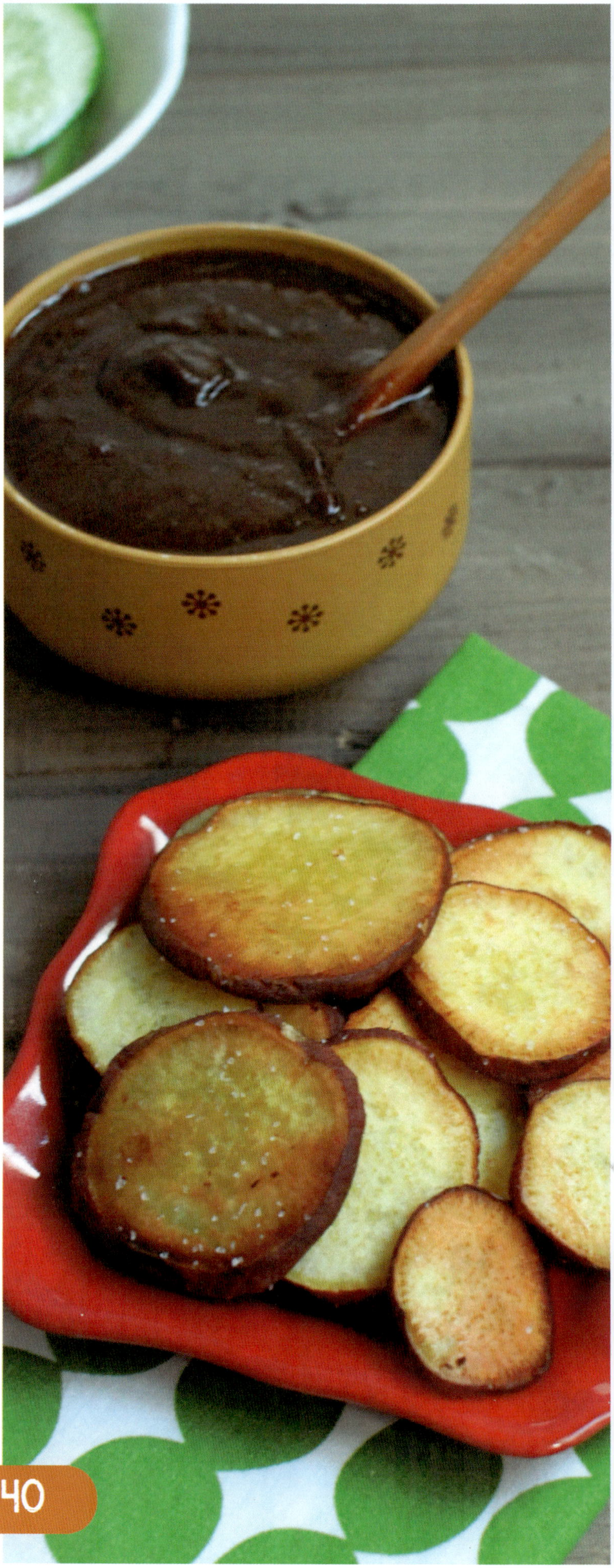

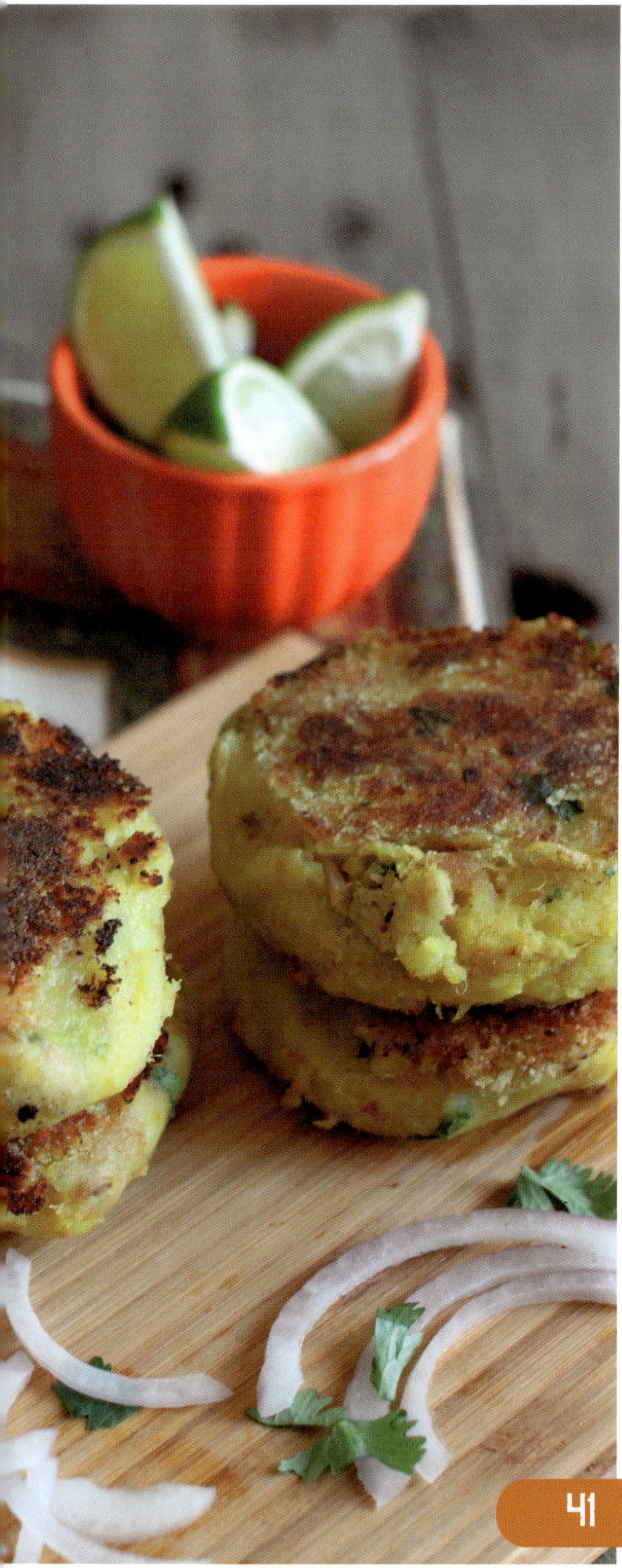

Fish Cutlets

Serves: 4   Time: 25 minutes

Ingredients:
- 2 medium white sweet potatoes
- 1 can (5 oz.) tuna - drained
- 1 small red onion - finely diced
- 1 TBSP fresh ginger - finely diced
- 2 cloves garlic - finely diced
- 5 curry leaves - finely diced
- 1/2 tsp pink salt
- 1/2 tsp turmeric powder
- 1 TBSP cilantro/ coriander leaves - chopped
- 2 TBSP cassava flour - for dusting
- 3- 4 TBSP coconut oil - for frying

Method:
- peel, chop and boil white sweet potatoes in a medium saucepan until fork tender
- while potatoes cook, finely diced the onion, garlic, ginger & curry leaves
- heat 1 TBSP coconut oil in a small saucepan, over medium heat and fry onion, garlic, ginger & curry leaves until soft and starting to brown. Once brown, remove from heat.
- when potatoes are cooked through, drain, return to hot pot and mash with a potato masher
- add onion mixture, a can of drained tuna and chopped cilantro to the potatoes and mix well
- use an ice-cream scoop to measure even cutlets and form in your hands into patties
- dust both sides of cutlets with cassava flour
- heat 3 TBSP coconut oil in a large skillet and fry for 2-3 minutes on each side until brown. Don't crowd the pan and cook in batches if necessary.

Great way to get more Omega-3 into your family's diet!

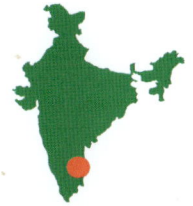

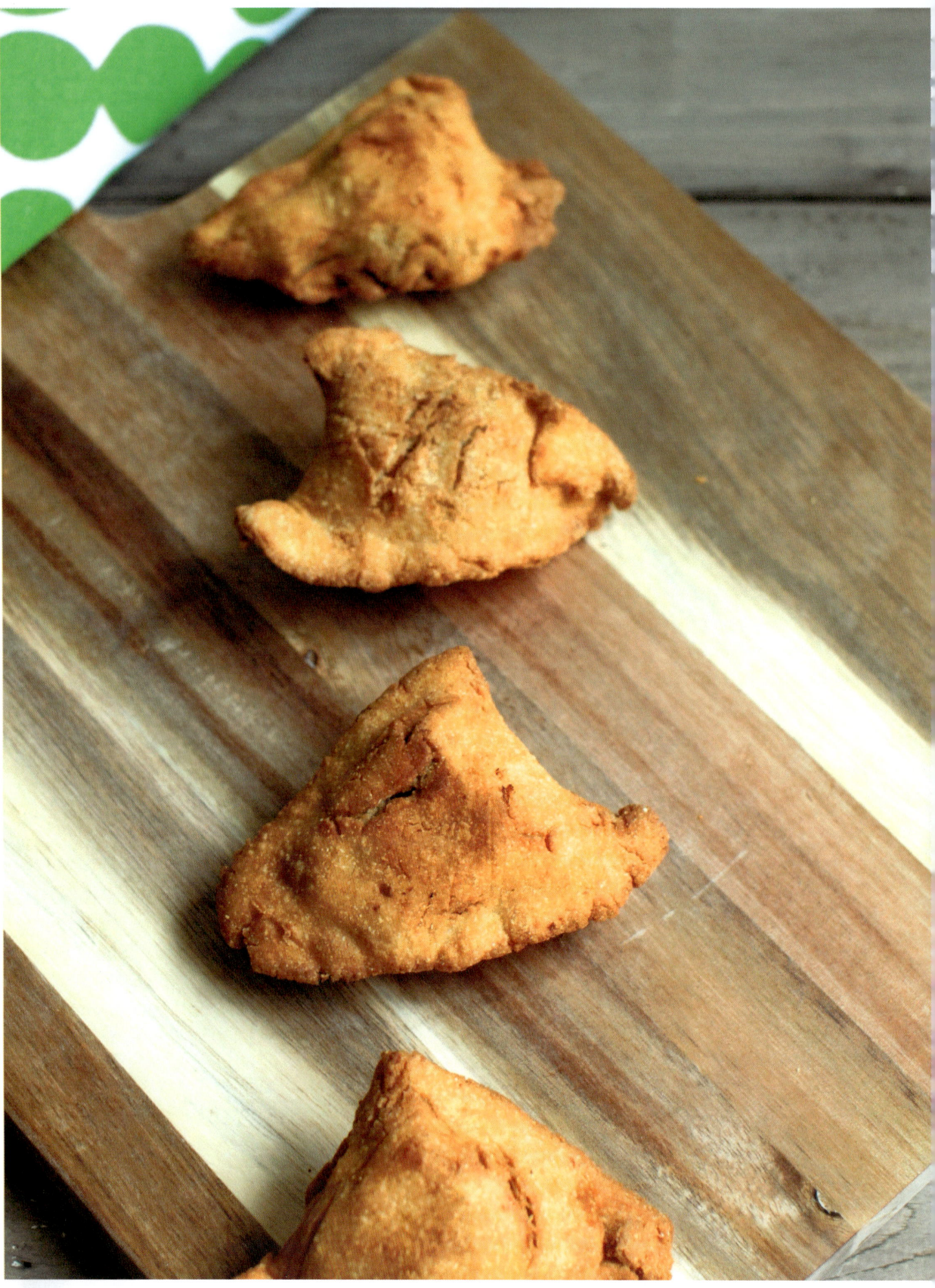

Sweet Potato & Beef
Punjabi Samosas

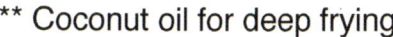

Makes: 12   Time: 55 minutes

Filling Ingredients:
- 1/2 TBSP olive oil
- 1/2 pound ground beef (or chicken)
- 1 small red onion - finely diced
- 1/2 TBSP dried ginger
- 1/2 tsp garlic powder
- 1/8 tsp mace
- 1/4 tsp turmeric
- 1/8 tsp sea salt
- 1/4 cup water
- 1/2 cup mashed sweet potatoes

Dough Ingredients:
- 2 cups cassava flour
- 1/2 tsp pink himalayan salt
- 1/4 cup coconut oil
- 1/2 cup + 2 TBSP warm water (+/-)

** Coconut oil for deep frying

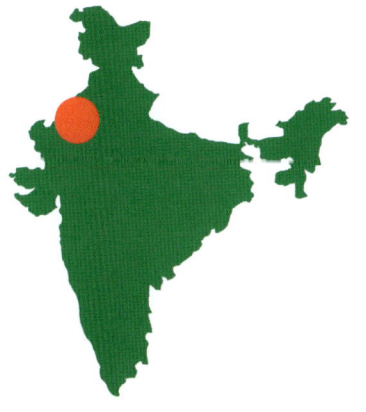

Reintroduction Note:
If you can eat seed spices, add 1/2 tsp cumin and 1/4 tsp coriander with the other spices.

Method:
- Make the dough - combine all ingredients except water and stir well, Slowly add water and knead until a smooth and non-sticky dough forms. Cover dough with a damp paper towel and allow to sit for 20 minutes
- Make the filling - heat olive oil in a skillet over medium heat, add ground beef and onion and sauté until meat is browned and onions are soft, add spices and water and cook until most of the water cooks off, remove from heat and add sweet potatoes and mix well to combine
- divide dough into 6 equal balls and keep them covered while working
- roll each ball between 2 pieces of parchment paper with a light dusting of cassava flour using a rolling pin until it forms a 6 inch circle
- Stuff Samosas - cut circle in half. Hold piece of dough in your hand and crimp the round edges together with fingers to form a cone. Fill with about 1 1/2 TBSP filling then use your fingers to crimp the top shut forming a triangle. Place stuffed samosas on a plate and cover with a dish towel for 20 minutes. *You will probably have some filling left...enjoy it for breakfast tomorrow.*
- Fry Samosas - heat about 2 cups coconut oil in a saucepan over medium heat until it bubbles when flour is sprinkled in. Use a slotted spoon to place 2-3 samosas at a time in the oil. Allow to fry over low to medium heat for 5-7 minutes until golden brown - turning several times during frying
- remove to a paper towel lined plate to drain and cool
- serve with mango chutney (pg. 32)

43

Indian Street Food Culture

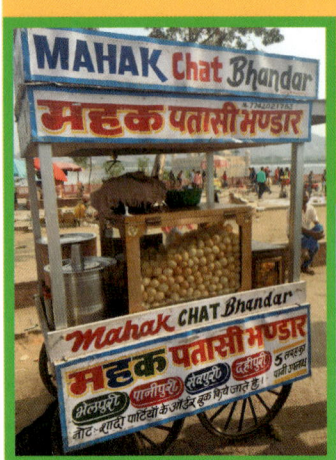

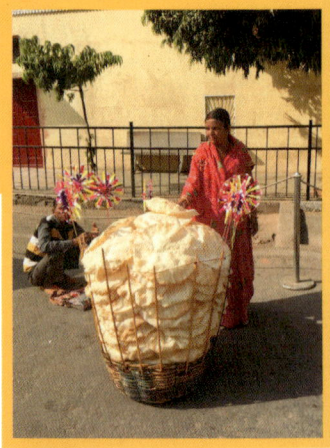

Street food is everywhere in India and it ranges from simple snacks like roasted lentils to dishes that could easily become a whole meal, like kebabs. The offerings that you'll find will vary by region just as the cuisine of the regions varies, but one sure thing is that you won't go hungry with the variety on every corner.

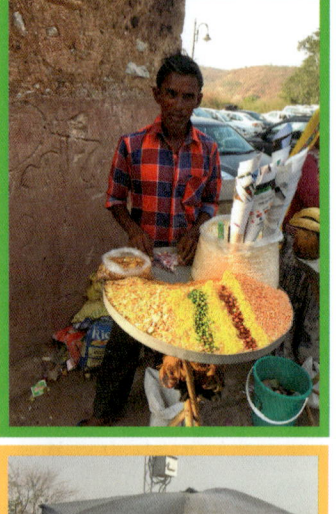

Many people rely on street food for much of their food while they're out during the day. My husband has even told me stories of his early days of working when he shared a small apartment with several other young men and how they survived on food from a local vendor most evenings.

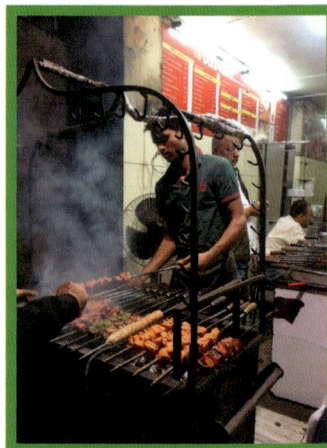

Street food is popular for it's taste and ease and is also popular as many people (especially young men) move away from home for work and long hours of work don't leave much time for cooking. So, why not walk down the street and pick up a some lime water, a samosa and some chaat, then finish it all off with a kulfi served out of a cloth wrapped clay pot to keep it chilled.

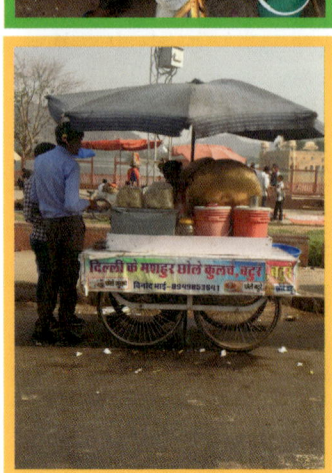

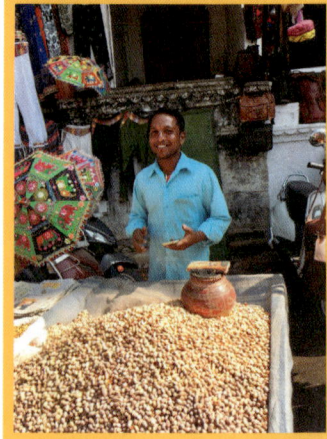

For a taste of Indian street food (AIP style), consider making:
- chaat - pg. 45
- plantain bajis - pg. 37
- reshmi kebab - pg. 62
- jal jeera - pg. 90
- mango kulfi - pg. 100

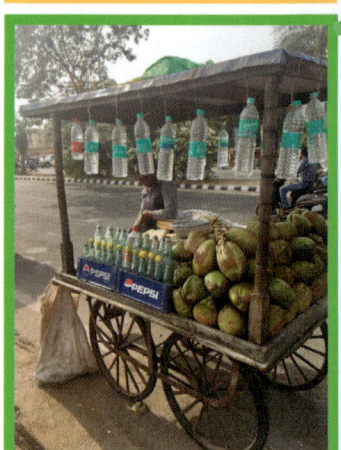

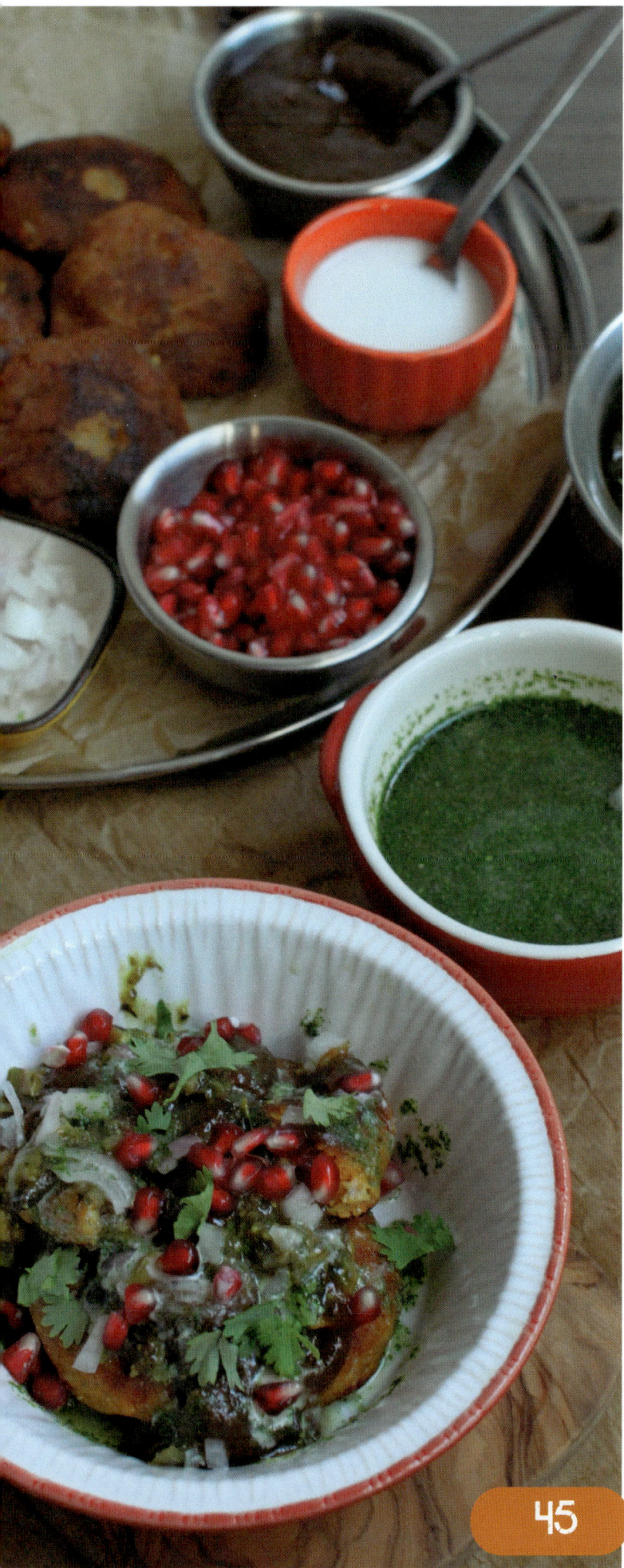

Delhi Style
Aloo Tikki Chaat

Serves: 3-4   Time: 55 minutes

Ingredients:
- 1 large sweet potato - about 3 cups chopped
- 1/4 tsp ginger powder
- 1/4 tsp garlic powder
- 1/4 tsp turmeric
- 1/2 tsp sea salt
- 1/4 tsp amchur powder
- 3/4 cup cassava flour
- coconut oil for shallow frying (2-3 TBSP)

Method:
- peel and boil potato in salted water until fork tender
- mash sweet potato with spices and cassava flour
- form into 10 patties about 3/4 inch thick and coat with cassava flour
- heat coconut oil in a skillet over medium heat
- fry in batches for 2-3 minutes on each side until golden brown

TO SERVE CHAAT:
- break 2 or 3 sweet potato patties into the bottom of a bowl
- top with a spoonful of mushroom masala, onion, pomegranate, cilantro and drizzles of coriander chutney, tamarind chutney and coconut cream

TOPPINGS:
- Mushroom Masala (pg. 85)
- Coriander Chutney (page 31)
- Date Tamarind Chutney (page 33)
- Diced Red Onion
- Chopped Cilantro
- Pomegranate Arils
- Coconut Cream or Yogurt

45

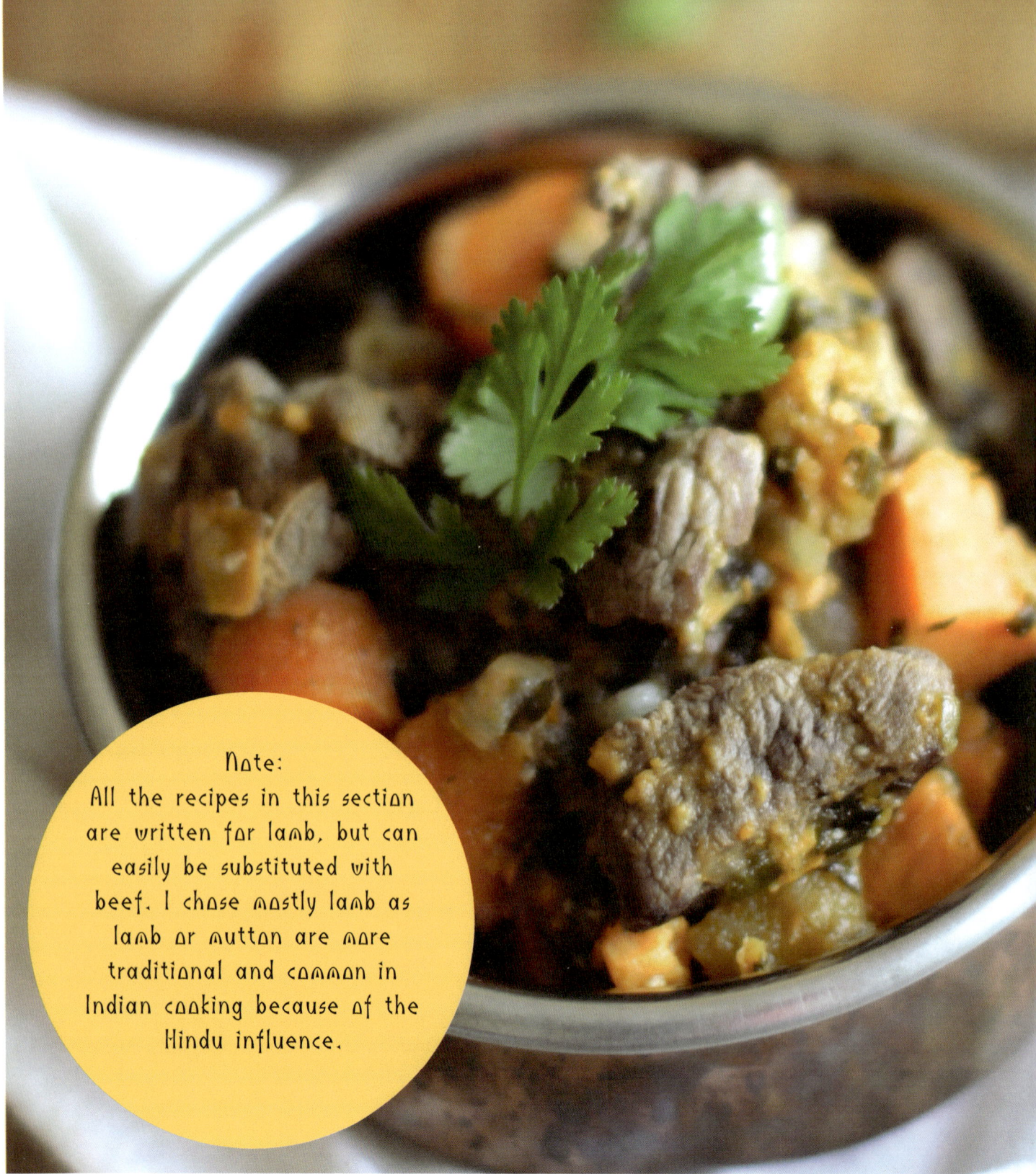

Non Veg: Lamb

Note:
All the recipes in this section are written for lamb, but can easily be substituted with beef. I chose mostly lamb as lamb or mutton are more traditional and common in Indian cooking because of the Hindu influence.

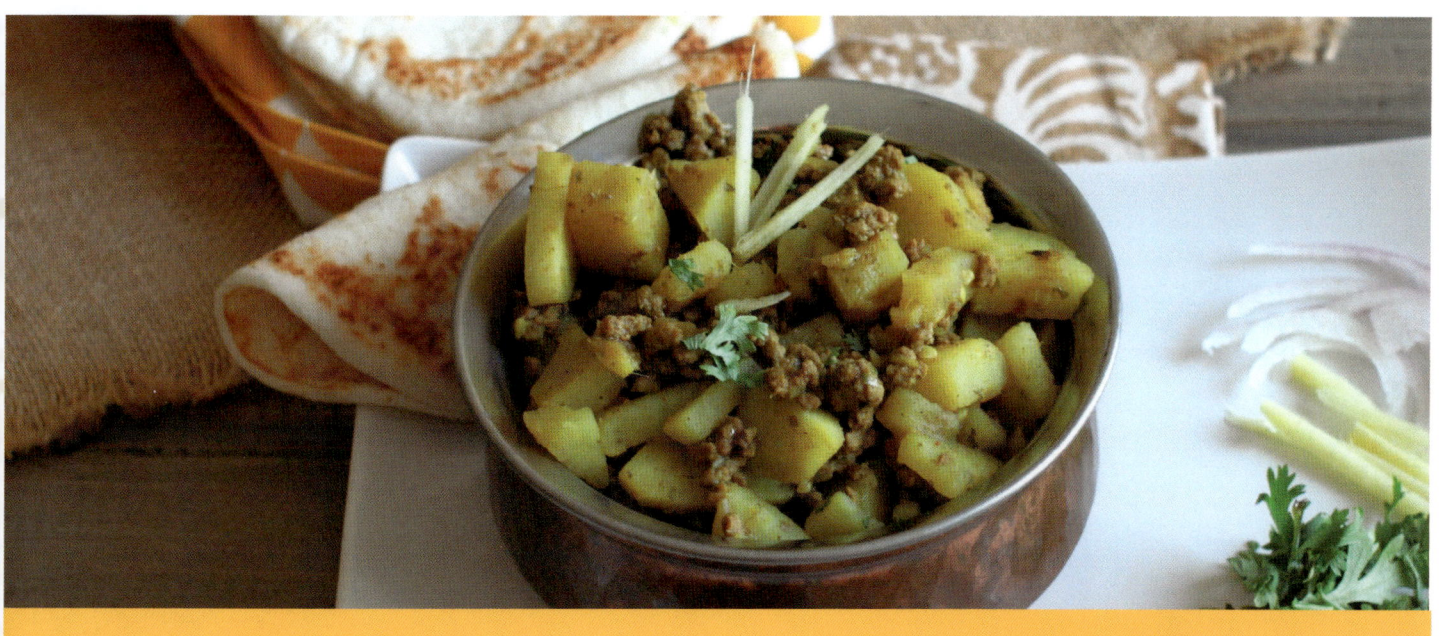

Lamb Aloo Keema

Serves: 4   Time: 35-40 minutes

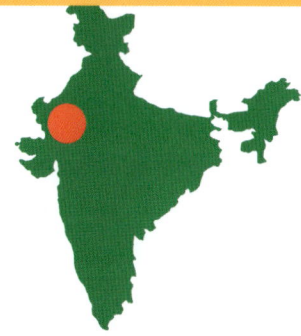

Ingredients:
- 1 red onion -finely diced
- 2 inch piece of ginger - finely diced
- 5 cloves garlic - finely diced
- 2 TBSP coconut oil
- 1 pound ground lamb
- 3/4 tsp pink himalayan salt
- 1/4 tsp cinnamon
- 1/8 tsp mace
- 1/8 tsp cloves
- 1/4 tsp ground ginger
- 3/4 tsp turmeric
- 2 tsp dried coriander leaves
- 2 medium white sweet potatoes - diced
- 3 cups water
- 2 TBSP coconut milk
- 3 TBSP fresh coriander leaves

Reintroduction Note:
If you can eat seed spices, add 2 tsp ground coriander and 1 tsp ground cumin with the other spices.

Method:
- prep ingredients : finely dice the onion, ginger and garlic
- heat coconut oil in a large skillet over a medium heat
- once oil is hot, add the lamb and allow it to begin to brown
- after about 3-4 minutes add the onion, ginger and garlic
- while lamb, onion, ginger and garlic cook, peel and diced the sweet potatoes and move to the side
- once lamb is cooked through and onions are browned, add all of the dry spices and stir well to combine. Allow lamb and spices to cook for 1-2 minutes until spices are fragrant
- add the diced sweet potatoes and water and reduce heat to low
- allow to simmer for about 15 minutes (stirring occasionally) until water is evaporated and potatoes are fork tender
- drizzle 2 TBSP coconut milk over top of the keema
- top with fresh coriander leaves
- serve with chapatis or cauliflower rice and mango chutney

Lamb Rogan Josh

Serves: 4   Time: 75 minutes

Ingredients:

- 1 pound lamb - cut into 1 inch cubes
- 2 TBSP coconut oil
- 1 medium red onion
- 1 medium carrot
- 8 cloves garlic
- 2 bay leaves
- 1/8 tsp clove powder
- 10 whole cloves
- 1 tsp pink himalayan salt
- 1 cinnamon stick - 4 inches
- 1/4 tsp cinnamon powder
- 1 TBSP ginger powder
- 1/4 cup fresh grated coconut
- 1 TBSP apple cider vinegar
- 1 cup water

This is winter comfort food at it's best!

Method:

- heat coconut oil in a pressure cooker or instant pot
- brown the lamb pieces in batches until all brown
- use a food processor to make a paste with the onion, garlic and carrot
- once all lamb is browned, add back to pot along with onion/ garlic/ carrot paste and stir to combine
- add all spices to the pot and sauté until spices are fragrant
- add coconut, vinegar and water to the pot
- place lid on pot and set to high pressure for 20 minutes
- allow steam to naturally release
- open pot and simmer out any remaining water
- serve with cauliflower rice or chapatis

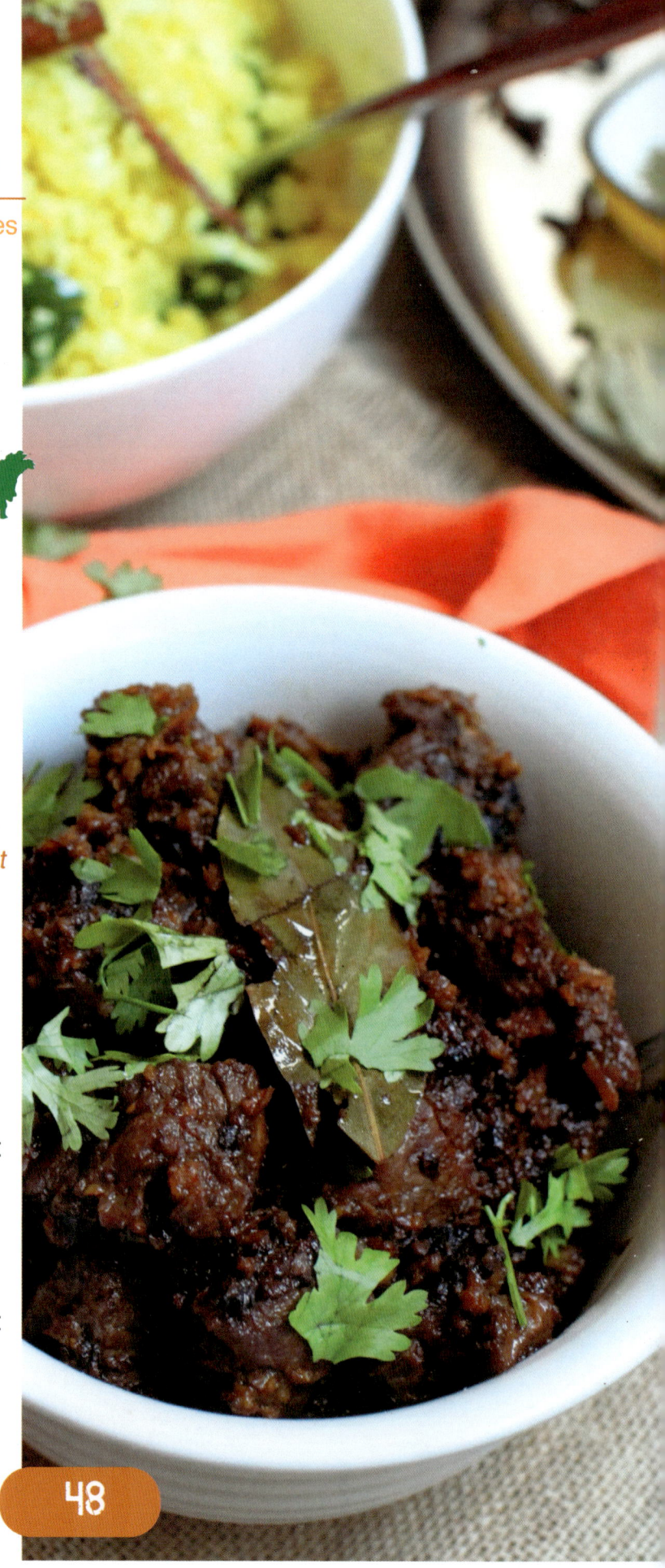

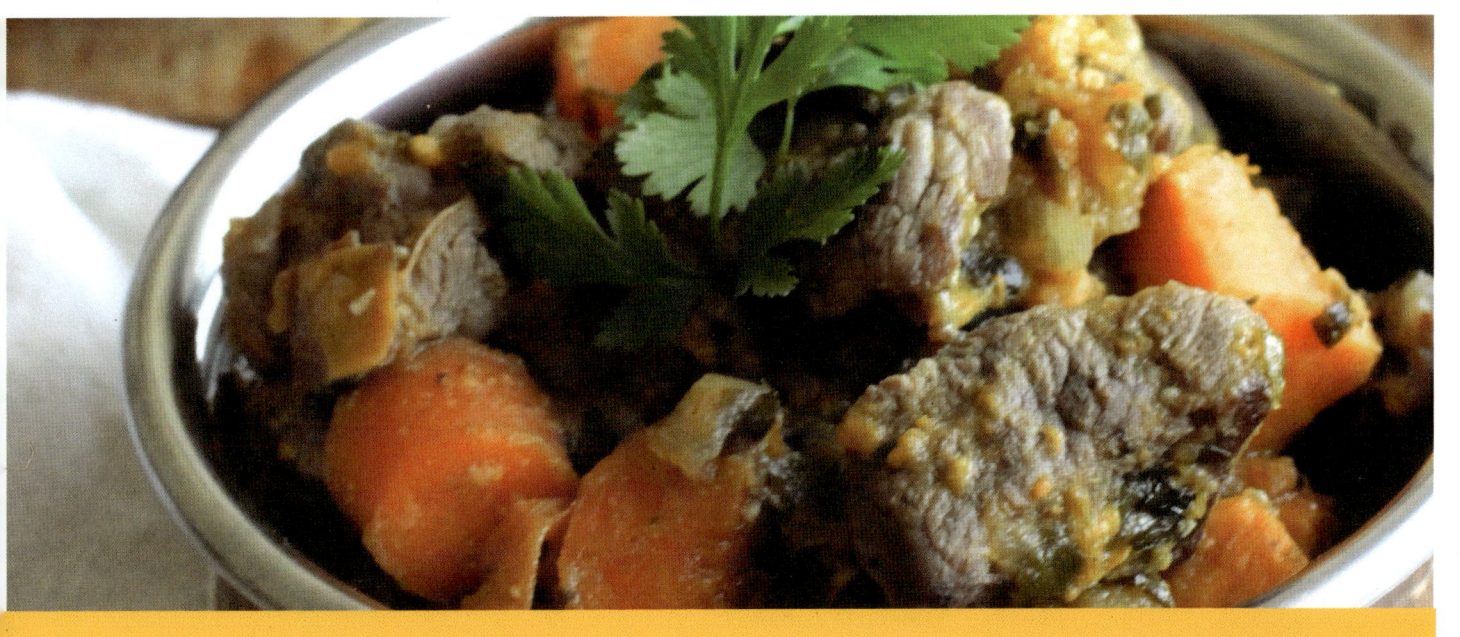

Lamb & Apricot Curry

Serves: 6-8   Time: 80 minutes

Ingredients:

Sauce
- 1 T olive oil
- 1 small white onion (diced)
- 5 cloves garlic - chopped
- 1 t dried turmeric
- 1 t sea salt
- 3 T fresh ginger - chopped
- 2 small carrots - chopped
- 1/4 cup chopped fresh cilantro
- 1 can coconut milk
- 2 cups broth
- 8 dried apricots - chopped
- Juice of 1 lime

Curry
- 1 T olive oil
- 2 pounds lamb
- 1 small onion - diced
- 1 medium sweet potato - chopped into large pieces (no need to peel)
- 2 carrots - chopped into large pieces
- 8 dried apricots (quartered)
- 1/2 cup frozen spinach

SERVING SUGGESTIONS:
Once cooked, serve with cauliflower or celeriac mash, cauliflower or plantain rice or with AIP Chapatis or Roti. Optional...top with shredded coconut, cilantro, raw onions, and/or raisins.

Method:

- - to make the sauce - heat oil in a small saucepan. Sauté the onions, then add ginger, garlic & spices. Allow spices to cook for a couple of minutes. Add remaining ingredients. Boil until carrots are tender (about 15 minutes). Blend well using an immersion blender.
- While sauce is boiling, brown lamb pieces & onion in olive oil in your pressure cooker.
- Add sweet potatoes, apricots, spinach and sauce to the pressure cooker
- *PRESSURE COOKER* - following your pot's instructions, bring to pressure and cook for 25 minutes.
- *STOVE TOP* - once all ingredients are together, allow to simmer for about an hour until meat is tender and sweet potatoes are falling apart
- *SLOW COOKER* - after browning meat & making sauce, combine all the ingredients in the slow cooker and cook on low for 7-8 hours

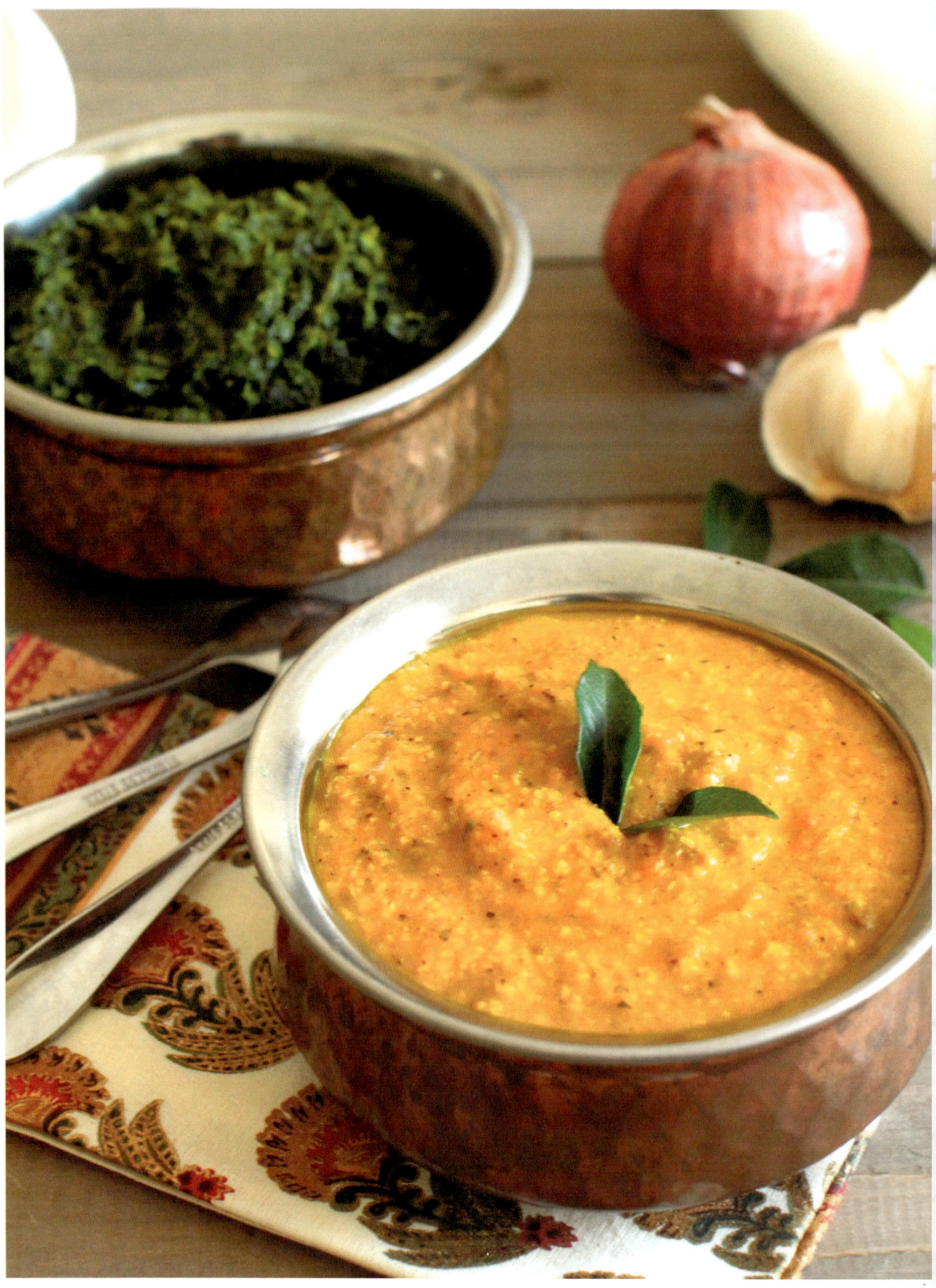

I'm sure you're wondering why the curry on the next page is called "Independence Curry"... so here's the story:

On the evening of August 14, I realized that the next day was Indian Independence Day. I wanted to do something special for my hubby, but had no idea what to do. When I asked him, his only comment was that he would like Indian food. I laughed to myself, because what is 'Indian food.' There were so many directions I could go and I honestly had no idea what would be the RIGHT dish to make for dinner. I scoured pinterest. I thought about things I'd made for him before, but nothing seemed right for a special dinner.

Then, I got to thinking about what I had made for 4th of July... I topped our perspective breakfasts with berries and other things in red, white and blue stripes. So, I started thinking about the Indian flag and what I could make to mimic the flag.

GREEN – no problem – spinach would do the trick

WHITE– again, no problem – we both handle white rice ok, so rice it was (you could easily sub cauliflower rice, mashed celeriac or even cassava)

ORANGE– hmm – can't really just serve carrots. So, I began to toss ingredients together and what came out what a perfectly orange and perfectly tasty lamb curry.

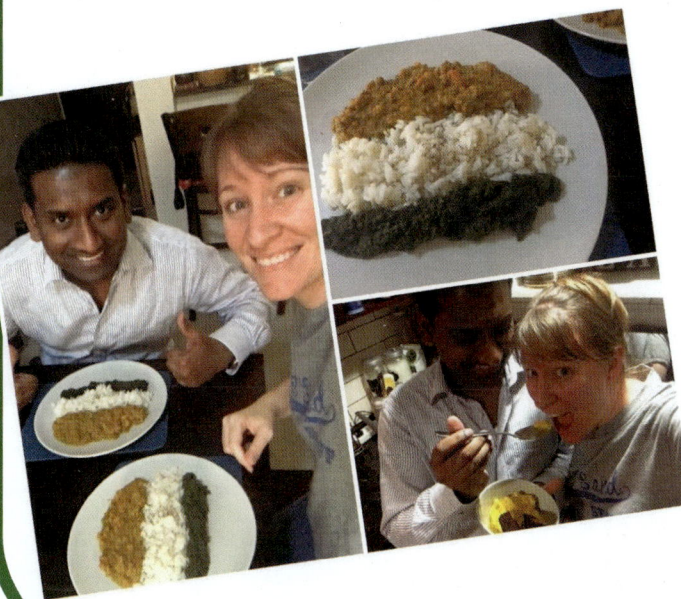

Here's some pics of us enjoying our dinner and the mango ice cream that we enjoyed for dessert.

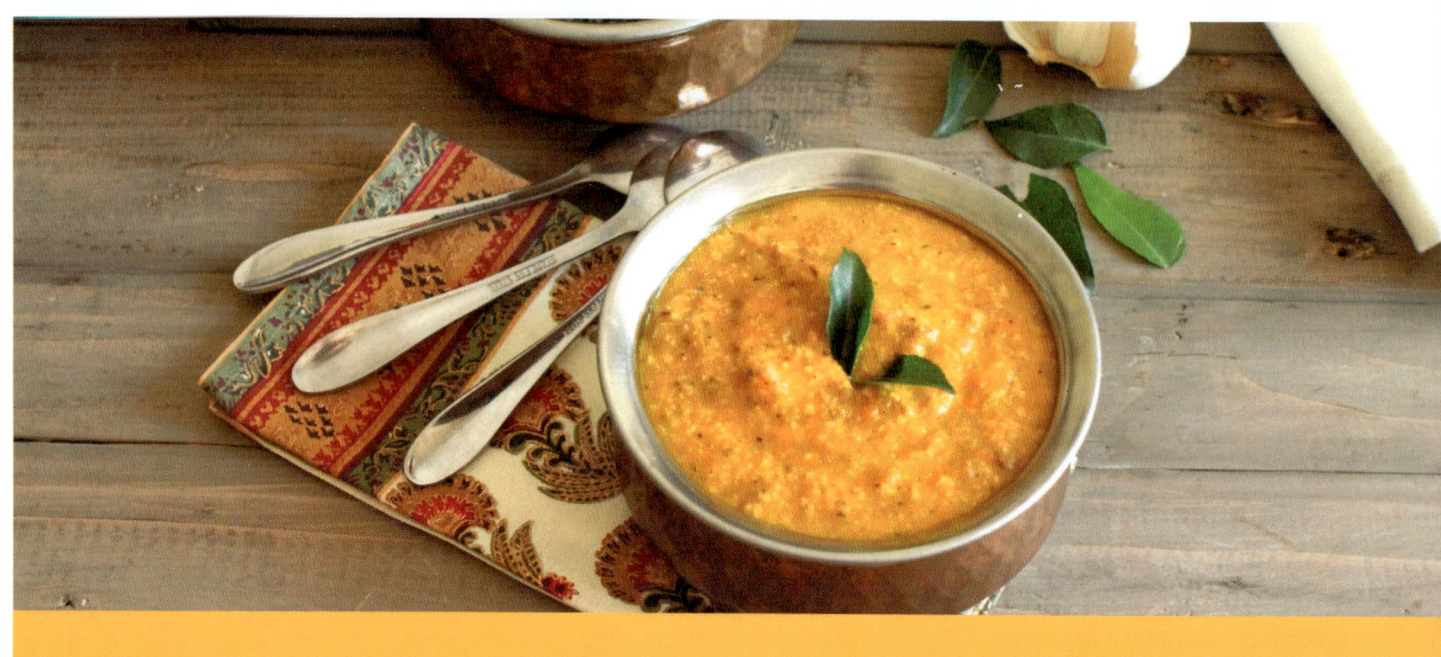

Independence Curry

Serves: 4-5   Time: 50 minutes

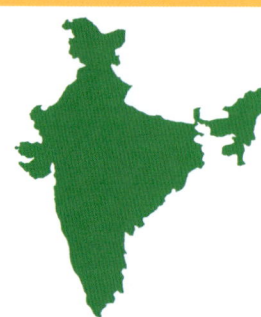

Ingredients:

LAMB
- 1 medium red onion
- 1 TBSP olive oil
- 1 pound ground lamb
- 1/2 tsp turmeric
- 1 tsp ground ginger
- 1/2 tsp pink salt

SAUCE
- 1 TBSP olive oil
- 2 red onions - rough chopped
- 2 inch piece of ginger
- 4 cloves garlic
- 12 curry leaves
- 1 tsp turmeric
- 2 tsp dried ginger
- 1/4 tsp cinnamon
- 1 TBSP dried coriander
- 2 cups fresh grated coconut
- 3 carrots
- 2 large green plantains
- 1/8 tsp pink himalayan salt
- 5 cups water

Method:

- finely dice a red onion
- heat 1 TBSP olive oil in a large stock pot over a medium heat
- once oil is hot, add onion, lamb, 1/2 tsp turmeric, 1 tsp ginger and 1/2 tsp salt and allow to cook until lamb is brown - about 8-9 minutes
- remove lamb to a bowl and set aside
- prep sauce ingredients: rough chop 2 red onions, peel and rough chop ginger, rough chop 4 cloves garlic, peel and cut carrots and plantains into 1 inch pieces
- add 1 TBSP olive oil back to the pan over medium heat
- once oil is hot, add onions, garlic, ginger, curry leaves and all dried spices - allow to cook over medium heat until onions are translucent and spices are fragrant - about 4-5 minutes
- add grated coconut and stir to absorb spices and all to cook together for 1 minute
- add carrots, plantains, water and salt and bring to a boil
- allow to simmer about 20 minutes until carrots and plantains are tender
- use an immersion blender to blend the sauce
- add lamb mixture back in and allow to simmer in the sauce for 5-10 minutes before serving
- serve with spinach (pg. 77) and cauliflower rice (pg. 28)

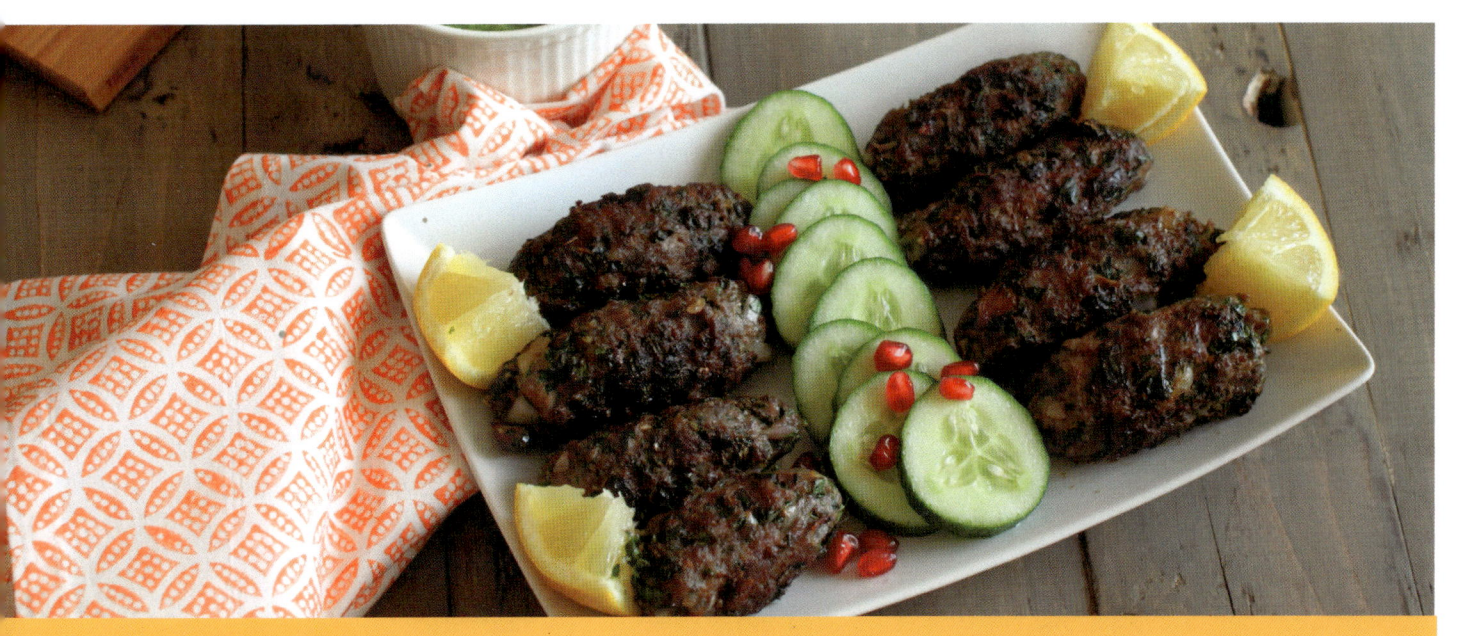

Spiced Lamb Kebabs

Serves: 3-4   Time: 25 minutes

Ingredients:

- 1 pound ground lamb
- 1 small red onion
- 4 cloves garlic
- 1 inch ginger
- small handful parsley
- small handful cilantro
- 2 TBSP chopped mint leaves
- 1/2 tsp sea salt
- 1/8 tsp mace
- 1/4 tsp turmeric
- 1/2 TBSP coconut oil

Method:

- rough chop the onion, garlic, ginger and herbs
- place everything except lamb in food processor and form a paste
- combine herb paste with lamb in a mixing bowl and mix well with your hands until seasonings are well combined
- heat a grill pan or skillet over a medium heat - add oil to pan when hot
- form lamb mixture into 8 sausage shapes by pressing them onto skewers
- cook about 3 minutes on each side in grill pan/ skillet (or on a grill if you have access to one - for the authentic street food taste)
- serve with coriander chutney, sliced cucumbers, a squeeze of lemon and a couple of roti for a full meal

TIP: Pack a couple of these, a roti, some cucumber slices and a small container of chutney or raita for a lunch that will make your coworkers jealous!

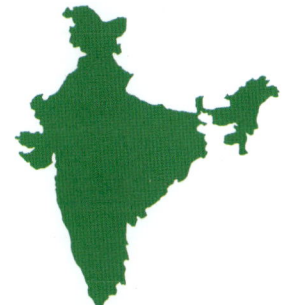

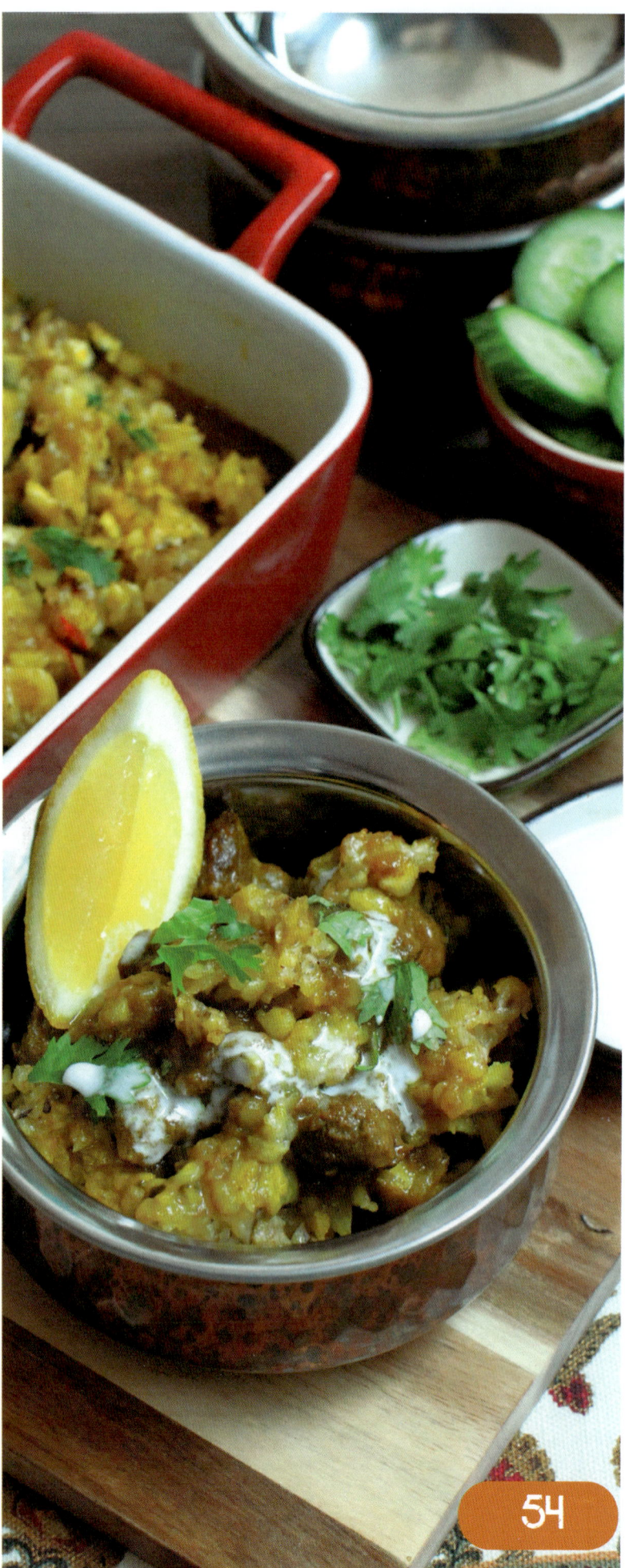

Lamb Biryani

Serves: 4 Time: 105 minutes

Ingredients:

TO MARINATE THE LAMB
- 1 pound lamb - cut into 1 inch cubes
- 1 tsp turmeric
- 3 TBSP coconut cream
- 1/4 tsp pink himalayan salt

TO COOK THE LAMB
- 4 TBSP coconut oil
- 1 bay leaf
- 8 cloves
- 3 inch piece of cinnamon (broken)
- 2 large red onions (sliced thin)
- 6 cloves of garlic (crushed)
- 2 inch pice of ginger (finely diced)
- pinch of saffron
- 1 tsp ginger powder
- 1/2 tsp mace
- 3/4 cup water

This biryani is well worth the time and effort it takes!

FOR THE 'RICE'
- 3 large green plantains
- 2 TBSP coconut oil
- 2 bay leaves
- 1/4 tsp cinnamon
- 1/4 tsp mace
- 1/2 tsp pink himalayan salt

TOPPINGS
- pinch of saffron soaked in 2 TBSP warm water
- 1/4 cup coconut cream
- 3 TBSP chopped cilantro
- lemon wedges

54

Method:

- start by marinating the lamb cubes by mixing 1 tsp turmeric, 3 TBSP coconut cream & 1/4 tsp pink himalayan salt and using it to coat the lamb. Place to the side for 20-30 minutes or in the fridge for a couple of hours
- place a pinch of saffron in 2 TBSP of hot water and set to the side to steep

COOK THE LAMB

- slice the onions thinly and finely dice or paste the garlic and ginger
- heat 4 TBSP coconut oil in a pressure cooker over medium heat or an instant pot set on sauté
- add whole spices and let them sizzle, then add the onions and cook for 10 minutes until starting to brown
- add the garlic and ginger and stir while cooking for 2 minutes
- add the powdered spices and allow to cook another 2 minutes
- add marinated lamb and allow to cook for 3-4 minutes to start to brown, then add 3/4 cup water and cook on high pressure for 18 minutes, quick release and allow to simmer for sauce to reduce by a third
- preheat oven to 350F

COOK THE RICE

- peel your plantains and either spiralize and cut into 'rice' sized pieces, or pulse in a food processor a few times until rice sized
- heat 2 TBSP coconut oil in a large skillet over medium heat
- add spices and allow to cook for 45 seconds before adding the riced plantains
- stir and cook for 5-6 minutes until all pieces start to turn golden brown. The starch will cause them to stick to the pan, but try to scrape up as much as possible as it adds to the flavor.

LAYER & BAKE THE DISH

- pour the lamb and sauce into the bottom of a baking dish
- top with the plantain rice. You may need to spoon it on top and then spread the rice out by hand to get it to cover all the lamb
- remove the saffron from the warm water and sprinkle the saffron water over the rice
- bake for 20 minutes
- top with chopped cilantro and serve with a drizzle of coconut cream and lemon wedges
- serve with fresh roti and a simple cucumber and onion salad and cucumber mint raitta (pg. 35)

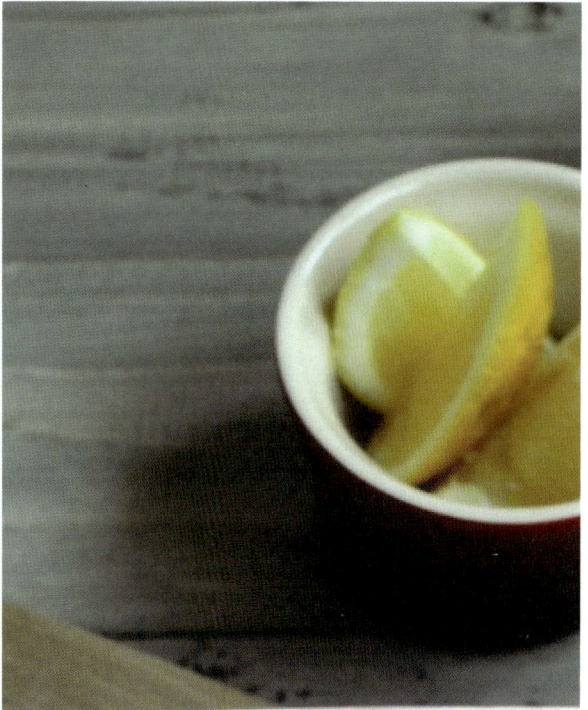

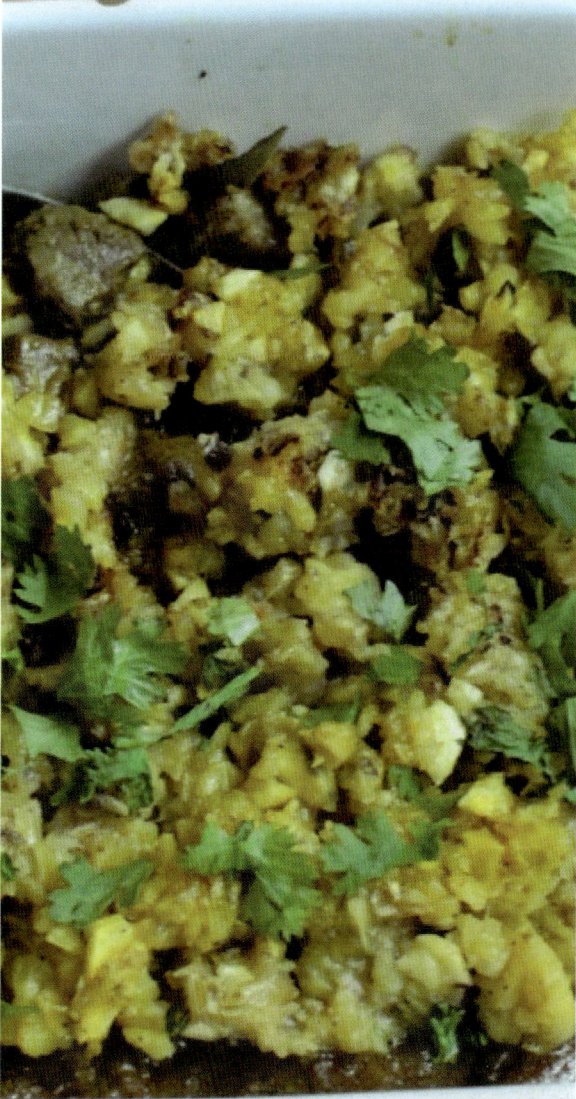

Curried Shepherd's Pie

Serves: 4-6   Time: 95 minutes

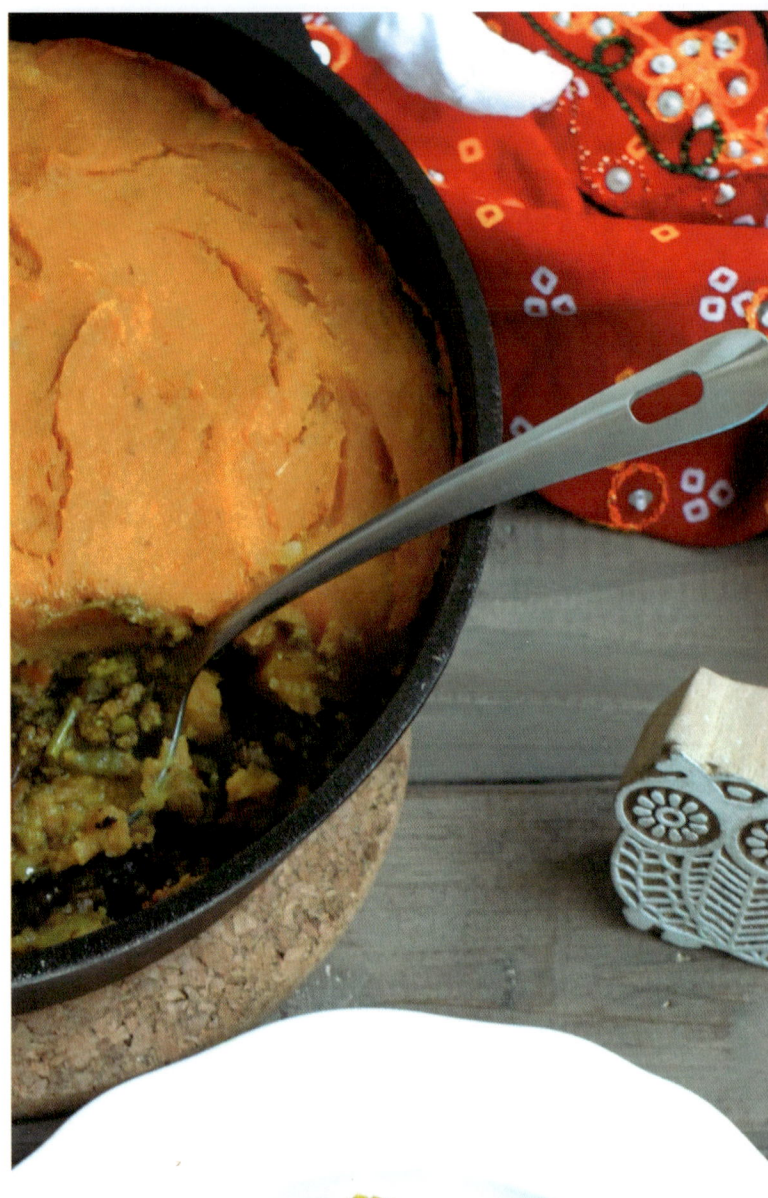

Ingredients:
- 2 medium/ large sweet potatoes
- 2 TBSP olive oil
- 5 curry leaves
- 2 TBSP ginger powder
- 2 tsp garlic flakes
- 2 tsp turmeric powder
- 1/8 tsp mace
- 1/8 tsp cloves
- 1/8 tsp cinnamon
- 1 1/4 tsp pink himalayan salt
- 1 pound ground lamb
- 2 TBSP dried fenugreek
- 1/4 cup raisins
- 3 medium carrots
- 2 medium turnips
- 1 cup chopped mushrooms
- 1 cup chopped asparagus *(or green beans if reintroduced)*

(Total 5 cups of chopped veggies of choice)

Method:
- chop sweet potatoes into bit sized pieces and boil until fork tender
- while potatoes boil...preheat oven to 375 F
- chop veggies into small dice
- in a large skillet heat olive oil and once hot add onions and spices and fry for 2-3 minutes
- add ground lamb and cook until no longer pink
- add raisins, carrots, turnips and mushrooms and cook for 10 minutes
- add asparagus
- drain sweet potatoes and puree with 1/2 tsp salt 1 tsp olive oil
- fill casserole dish with lamb mixture and top with sweet potatoes
- bake uncovered for 45 - 50 minutes

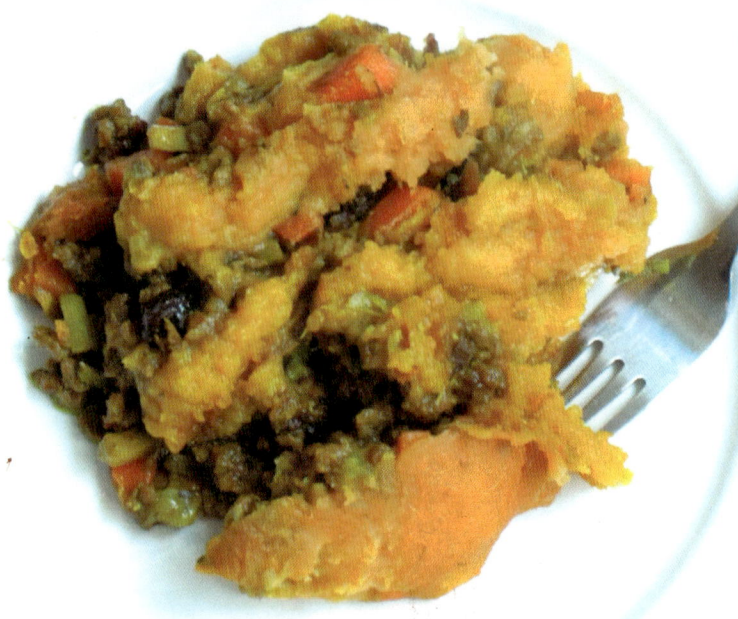

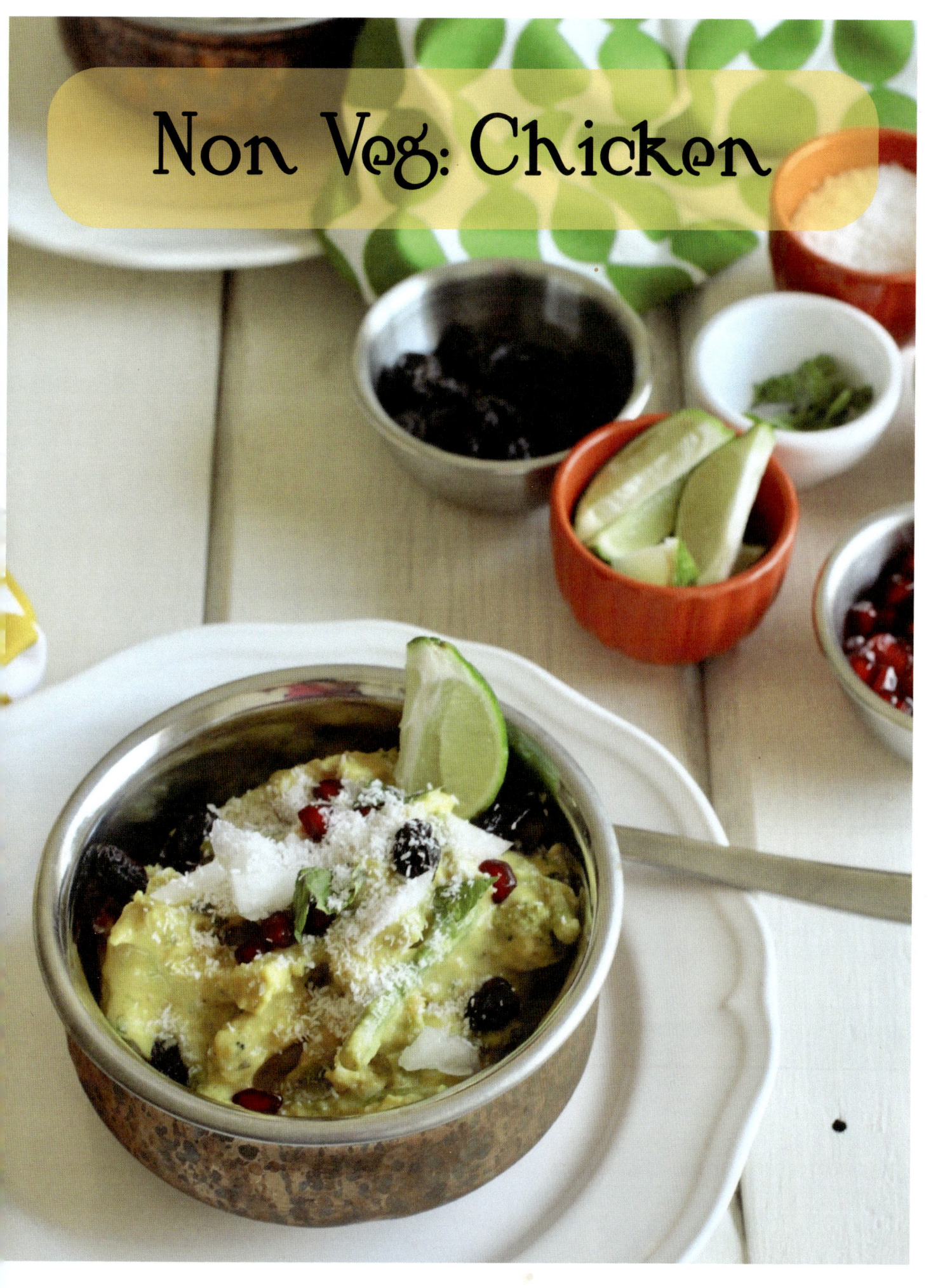

Non Veg: Chicken

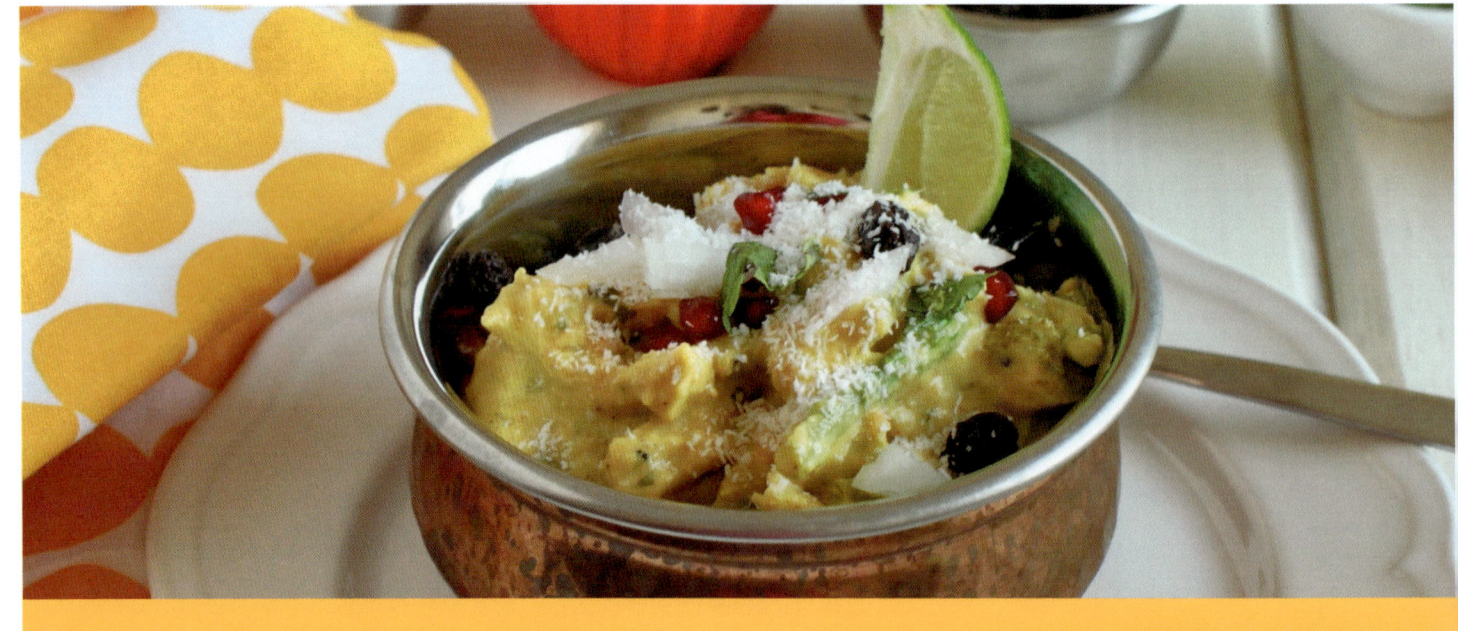

Brakenhurst Chicken Curry

Serves: 4-6   Time: 55 minutes

Ingredients:
- 1 Tablespoon olive oil
- 1 large red onion - chopped
- 2 carrots - chopped
- 1/3 of a daikon (or 1/2 cup radishes) - chopped
- 1.5 tsp pink himalayan salt
- 1/2 tsp ground cinnamon
- 1 TBSP garlic flakes
- 2 inch piece of ginger - peeled and chopped finely (or grated)
- 1 TBSP dried ginger powder
- 1 tsp turmeric powder
- 1 can of coconut milk
- 6 cups of chopped veggies - broccoli, asparagus, butternut, cauliflower - bite sized pieces
- 1 pound chicken - poached/roasted
- 1/4 cup chopped parsley
- Juice of 1 lime

Method:
- heat olive oil in a large soup pot over medium heat
- add chopped onion and sauté for 3-4 minutes
- add carrot & daikon (or radishes) and continue cooking for a few minutes
- add salt, cinnamon, garlic ginger (fresh & dried) and turmeric and allow to cook until you smell the spices (2 minutes)
- add enough water to cover the veggies and simmer until the carrots and daikon are soft (15 minutes)
- *This recipe is a great way to use a chicken you roasted earlier in the week..or even a clean rotisserie chicken.... or simply poach a few chicken breasts.*
- once veggies are soft, add coconut milk and use an immersion blender to blend until smooth. Make sure you get all the little ginger pieces (no one wants to bite down on one of those)
- add 6 cups of vegetables *(broccoli & asparagus is my favorite combo... also good with pumpkin, butternut & carrots.... and have used butternut, asparagus and cauliflower).... great way to clean out the produce drawer* and allow veggies to cook until tender (depends on the veggie - but probably 10-15 minutes.
- add cooked chicken about 5 minutes before veggies are ready
- after cooking is finished, stir in chopped parsley and the juice of a lime.

58

Seafood/ Fish Variation:

If you want to make a seafood variation...

(1) make the sauce as is, except only the fresh ginger and no daikon
(2) use heartier vegetables to balance out the lightness of the seafood - pumpkin, sweet potato, broccoli all work
(3) use 1/4 cup cilantro at the end instead of parsley and the juice of 2 lemons
(4) add raw seafood to the cooked sauce & veggies and allow to cook in the sauce - just a few minutes
(5) the best toppings are the more tropical ones - pineapple, mango, herbs & coconut

---

AIP Topping Options:

- toasted coconut
- raisins
- pomegranate arils
- fresh mint
- fresh parsley
- fresh cilantro
- chopped pineapple

- sliced banana
- chopped mango
- lime wedges
- diced spring onions
- chopped red onions
- date tamarind chutney (pg. 34)
- mango chutney (pg. 32)

This chicken curry is based on an 'Indian' dish that we used to enjoy in Kenya and is my go-to holiday meal.

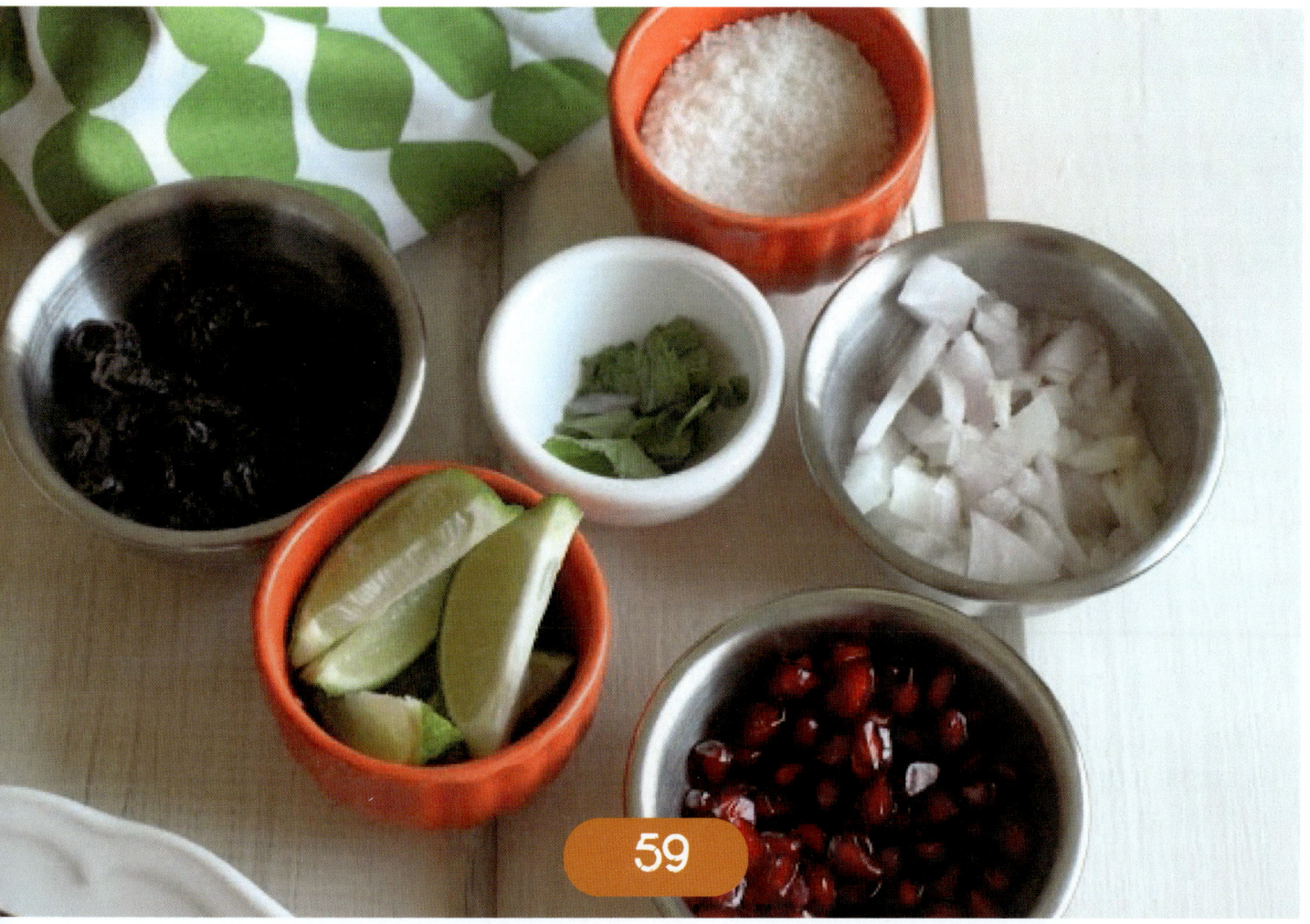

59

Goan Chicken Xacuti

Serves: 4   Time: 50 minutes

Ingredients:
- 2 TBSP olive oil
- 1 large or 2 small red onions
- 6 cloves garlic
- 2 inch piece of ginger
- 1 tsp tamarind paste
- 1 1/2 cups shredded coconut (fresh if possible)
- 1/4 tsp cloves
- 1/4 tsp mace
- 1 tsp cinnamon
- 1/2 tsp turmeric powder
- 1 tsp ginger powder
- 1/2 tsp sea salt
- 1 pound chicken breasts or thighs (cut into bite sized pieces)
- 1 1/2 1/2 cup water

Method:
- heat olive oil over a medium heat in a large pot
- rough chop onion, garlic and ginger
- add onion to hot oil and cook until starting to brown
- while onion is browning, cut 1 pound of chicken into bite sized pieces
- once onion is starting to brown, add ginger and garlic and cook another 3 minutes
- add tamarind, coconut and all the spices and fry until coconut is starting to brown
- add 1/2 cup water and use it to scrape all the browned bits off the bottom of the pan and allow to simmer for 5 minutes before using an immersion blender to puree the sauce
- add the chicken into the sauce and simmer for 20-25 minutes until chicken is cooked through
- serve with roti and kachumber salad (pg. 38)

Reintroduction Note:
If you can eat seed spices, add 1/2 tsp cumin seeds and a few mustard seeds with the onion.

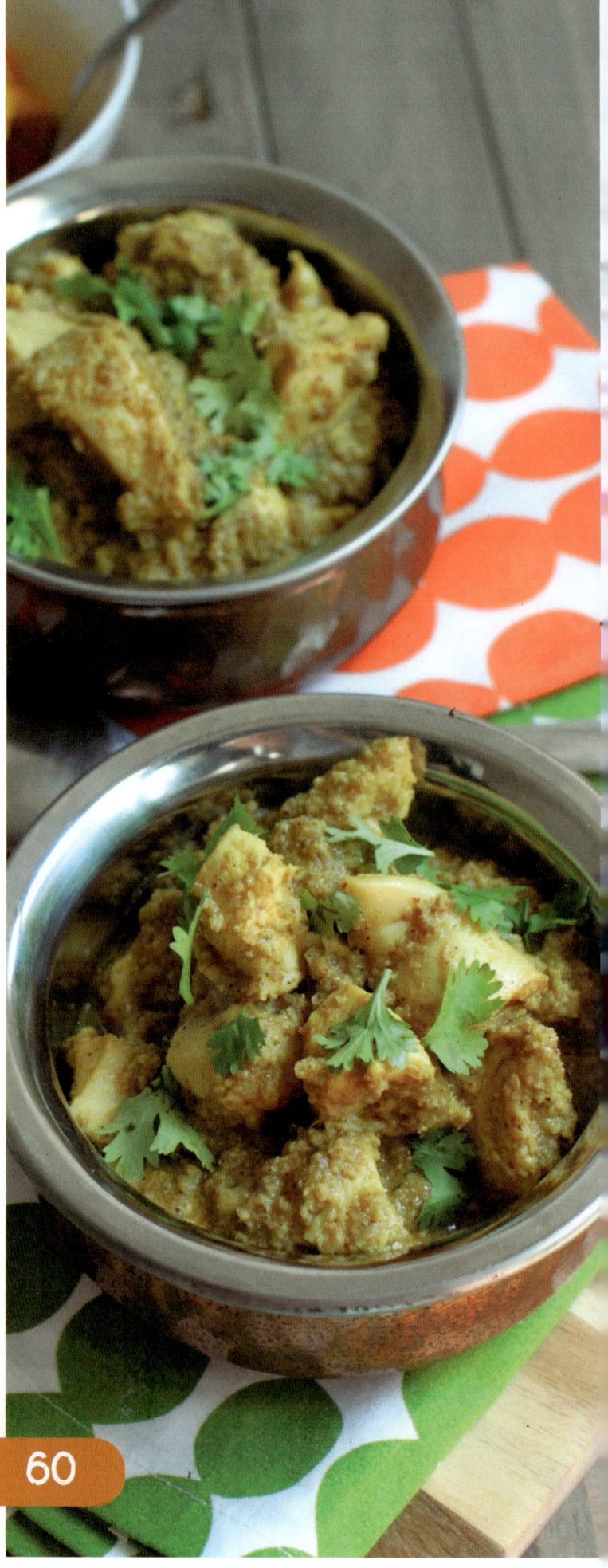

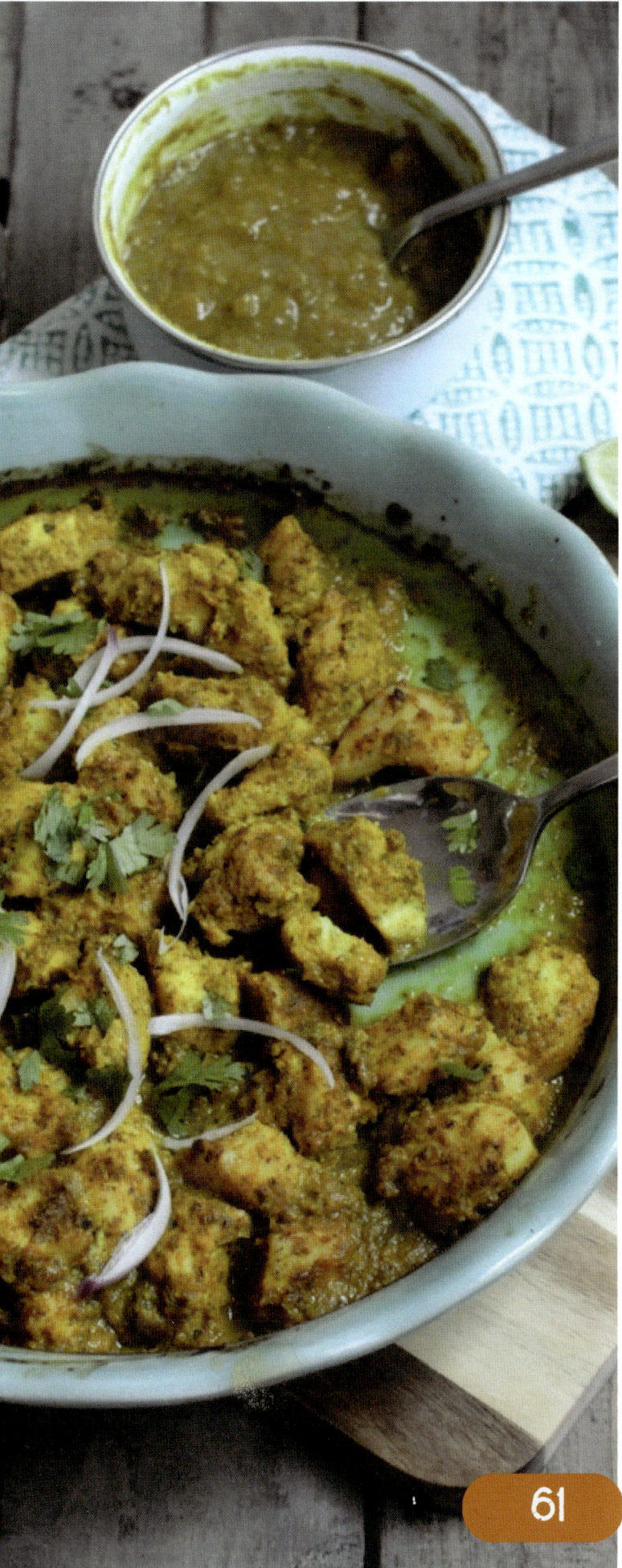

Chicken Tikka Masala

Serves: 4   Time: 50 minutes

Ingredients:
- 1 pound chicken breast - cut into 1 inch cubes
- 2 cloves garlic
- 1/2 red onion
- 2 inch piece of ginger
- 1/4 cup coconut milk
- juice of 2 limes
- 1 TBSP dried coriander leaves
- 2 tsp turmeric powder
- 1 tsp ginger powder
- 1/8 tsp cloves
- 1/8 tsp cinnamon
- 1/2 tsp pink himalayan salt
- 1 TBSP fresh coriander leaves chopped

Method:
- preheat oven to 400 F/ 200 C
- cut chicken into 1 inch cubes and place in a baking dish
- place all remaining ingredients in a food processor and process until a smooth paste is formed
- *(if your coconut milk is thick - add 1/2 TBSP water to the paste)*
- spoon the paste over the chicken and stir until all the chicken is coated
- bake at 400 F for 30 minutes, then turn on the broiler and broil/ grill for 5 minutes to brown the top
- serve with mango chutney (pg. 32) and cassava thoran (pg. 76)

Reintroduction Note:
If you can eat seed spices, add 1/2 tsp each of cumin powder and coriander powder with the other spices.

Chicken Reshmi Kebabs

Serves: 4   Time: 50 minutes

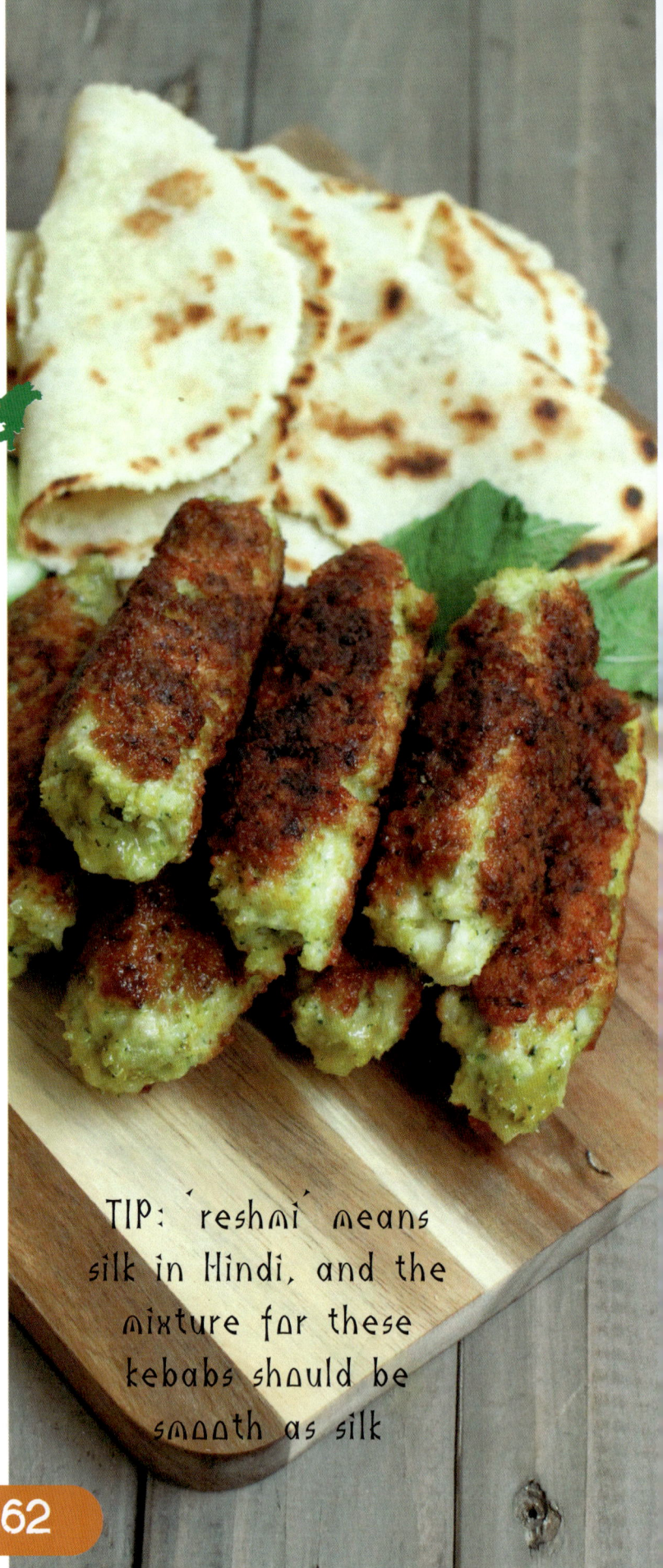

Ingredients:
- 1 small red onion
- 2 garlic cloves
- handful of cilantro leaves
- 1/4 cup plantain chips
- 1 tsp pink himalayan salt
- 1/2 tsp turmeric
- 1/4 tsp mace
- 1 tsp ginger powder
- 1 pound ground chicken (or chicken breasts cut into cubes)
- 2 TBSP coconut cream

- 1 TBSP coconut oil for cooking

Method:
- place rough chopped onion and garlic and cilantro in a food processor bowl and pulse until a smooth paste starts to form
- add plantain chips and pulse until chips turn to crumbs
- add spices, chicken and coconut cream and process until all ingredients are well combined and chicken is finely ground. If your chicken was pre-ground, this should just take a few pulses
- divide chicken mixture into 8 pieces and form around skewers and place in fridge for 20 minutes
- heat oil in a large skillet over a medium heat and cook kebabs for about 4 minutes in each side
- serve with roti (pg. 22) and kachumber salad (pg. 38)

TIP: 'reshmi' means silk in Hindi, and the mixture for these kebabs should be smooth as silk

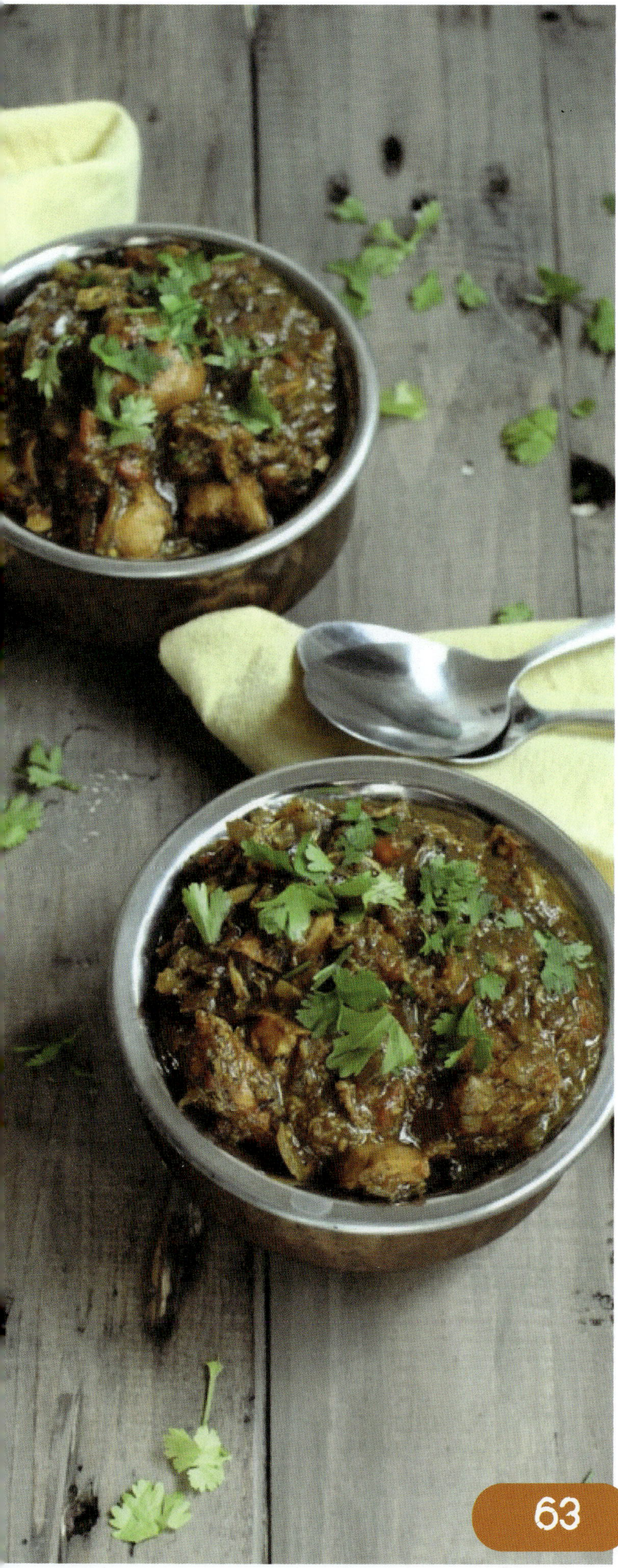

Chicken Chettinad Curry

Serves: 4   Time: 55 minutes

Ingredients:

- 1 pound of chicken breast or thighs
- 1 tsp turmeric
- juice of 1 lemon
- 1 tsp pink himalayan salt
- 1/2 cup shredded coconut
- 3 TBSP olive oil
- 3 medium red onions
- 2 inch piece of ginger
- 1 TBSP garlic granules
- 12 curry leaves
- 1 tsp cinnamon
- 1/2 tsp mace
- 1/2 tsp cloves
- 1 TBSP dried ginger
- 1 carrot
- 2 TBSP tamarind chutney (pg. 34)
- 1/4 cup cranberries
- 1 cup water

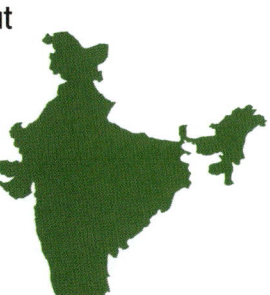

Method:

- cut chicken into bite sized pieces and marinate chicken in turmeric, lemon juice and 1/2 tsp salt
- toast coconut in a dry pan over a medium heat for 45 seconds until golden brown & set aside
- heat olive oil in large pot or pressure cooker (instant pot)
- thinly slice onions and chop ginger
- sauté onions and ginger for 6-8 minutes
- add curry leaves and other spices and cook for another 2 minutes
- finely dice carrot and add carrot, cranberries, chutney, water, toasted coconut and chicken to the pot
- simmer for 45 minutes or pressure cook for 20 minutes (quick release pressure)
- serve with cassava thoran, roti or cauliflower rice

63

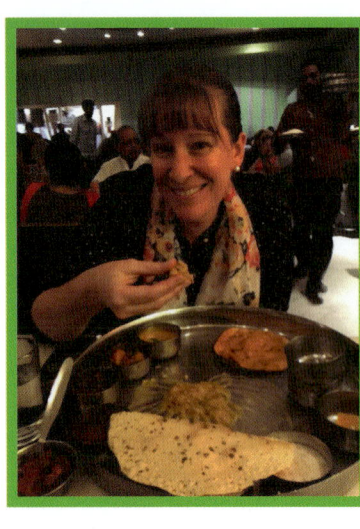

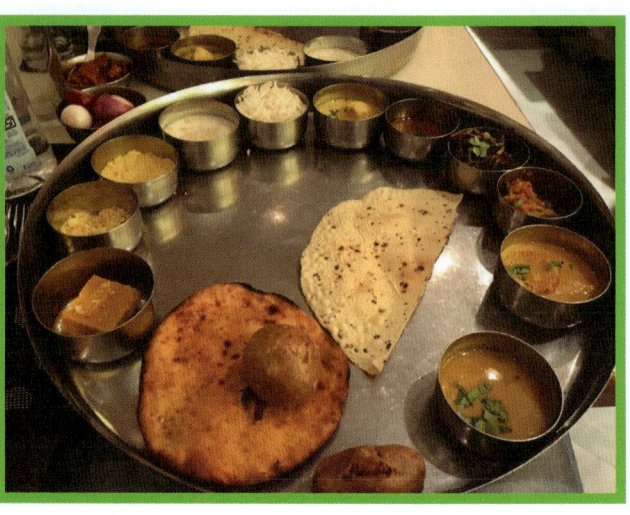

Thali

My favorite way to enjoy Indian food is in the form of a Thali. The literal definition of thali is plate - talking about the platter (often a metal tray) that the meal is served on. And a thali is a set menu often served in Indian restaurants comprised of 8-15 dishes all served on a round platter. Thalis vary by region and can either be all veg dishes or can be comprised of meat or seafood dishes. Typically a thali would include rice, dal, roti, veg and/ or meat dishes, yogurt, chutney or pickle, and a sweet.

Serving a thali would be a great way to expose your family and friends to a variety of Indian dishes all in one setting. If I were creating a thali from the recipes in this book, I would include:
- garlic cilantro roti - pg. 23
- coconut turmeric rice - pg. 28
- yellow dal - pg. 86
- cabbage thoran - pg. 75
- mango curry - pg. 81
- simple saag - pg. 77
- gajar methi sabzi - pg. 84
- prawn masala - pg. 67
- kerala fish molee - pg. 71
- cucumber mint raitta - pg. 35
- sweet potato gulab jamun - pg. 99

Check us out with our fun Rajasthani hats while enjoying thali in Jaipur!

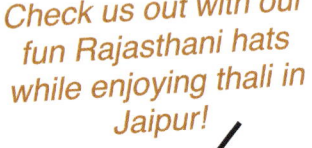

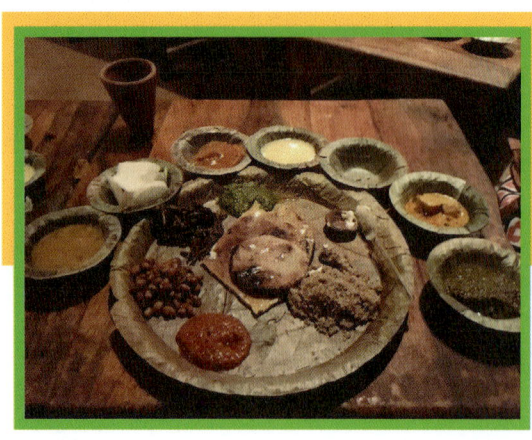

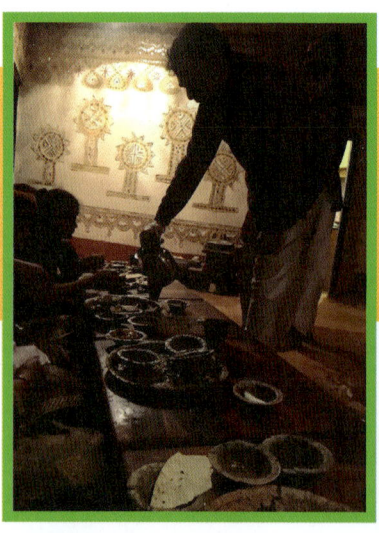

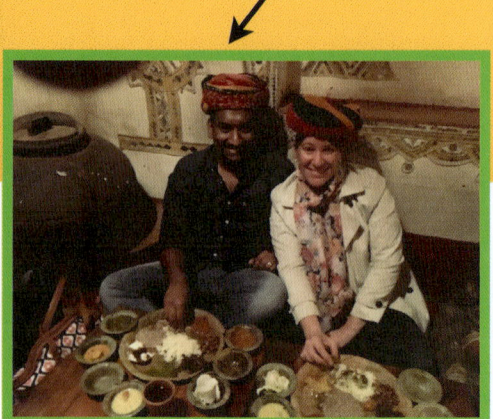

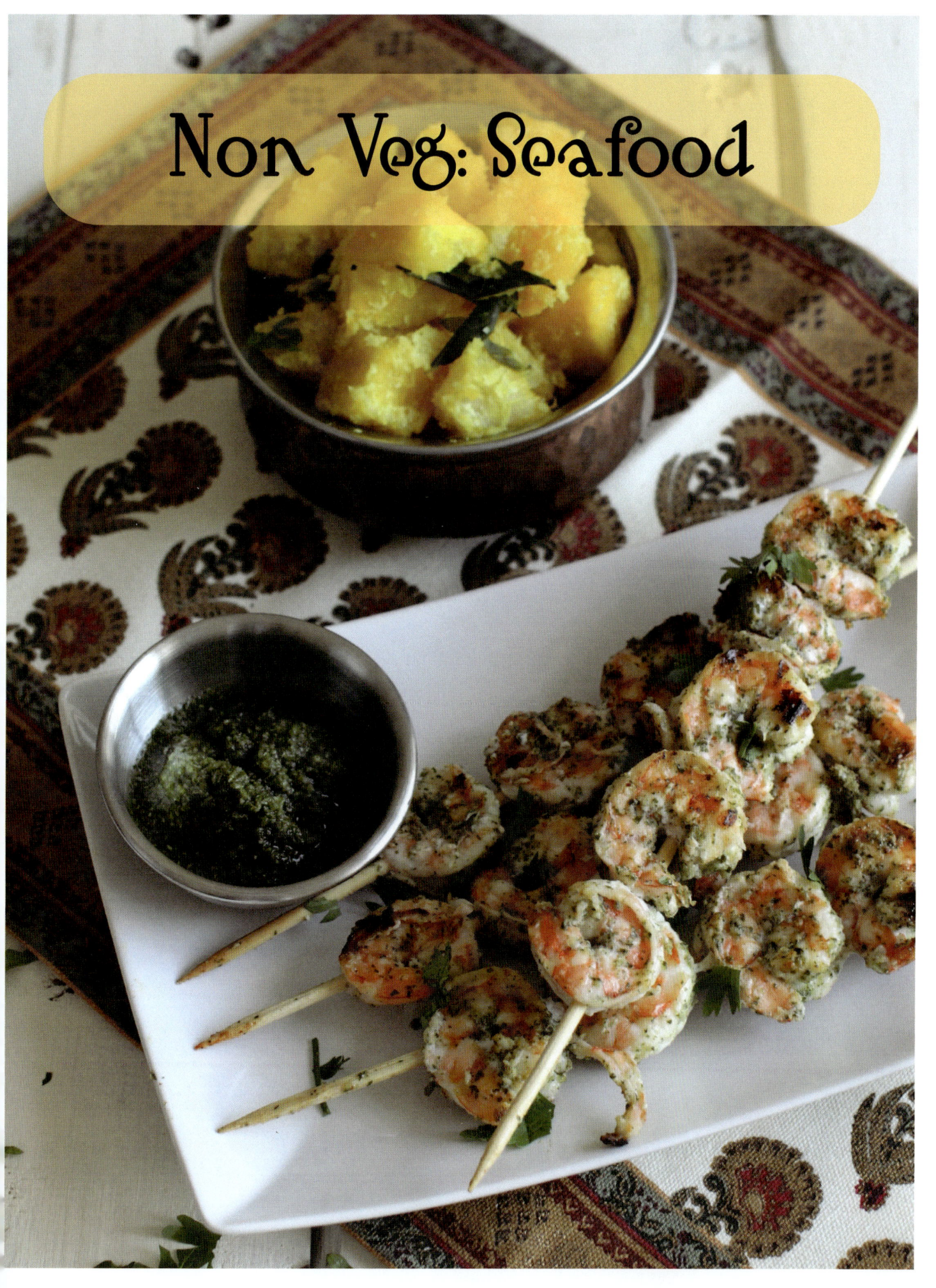

Non Veg: Seafood

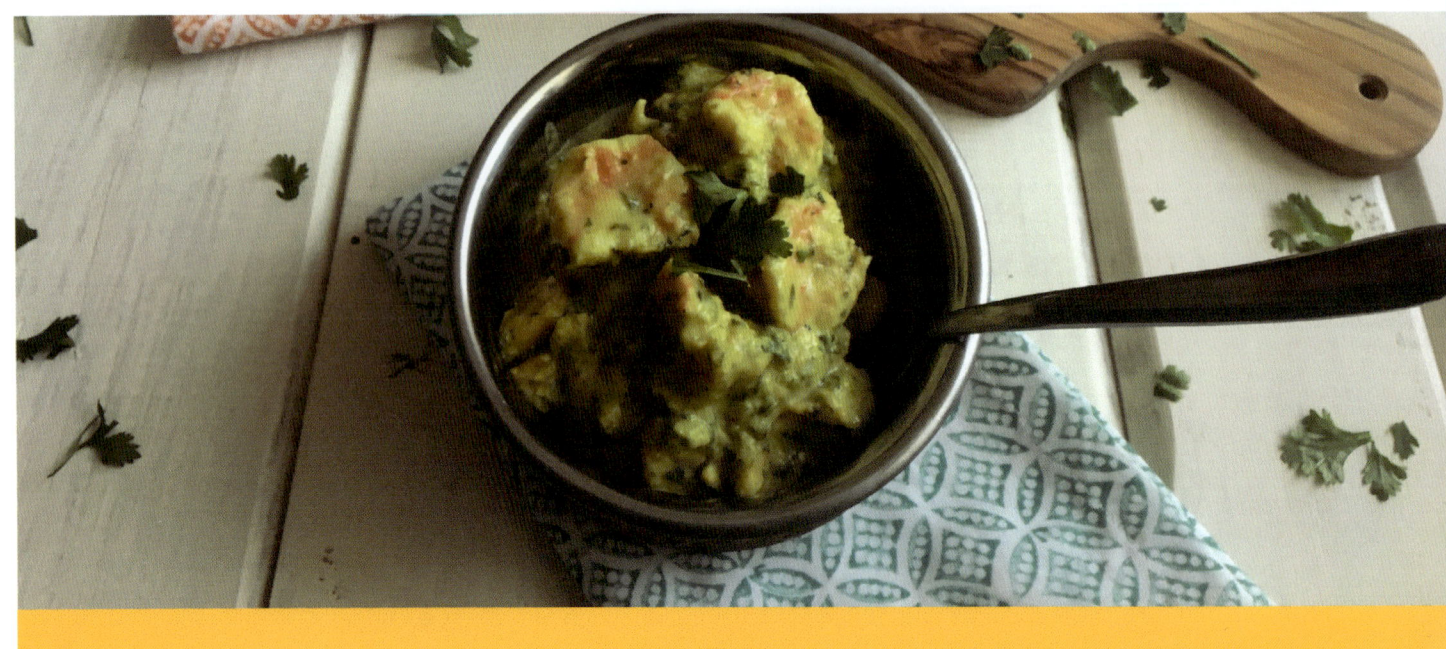

Shrimp & Sweet Potato Coconut Curry

Serves: 4-5   Time: 30 minutes

Ingredients:
- 1 TBSP olive oil
- 1 large white onion- diced
- 1 inch piece of fresh ginger - grated
- 1 TBSP garlic granules
- 1 TBSP dried ginger powder
- 1 TBSP dried cilantro leaves
- 1/2 TBSP turmeric powder
- 1 1/2 t sea salt
- 1 large or 2 medium sweet potatoes - cut into 2 inch chunks
- 1 cup frozen spinach
- 3 cups water (or fish stock)
- 1 1/2 pounds cleaned shrimp
- 1 cup coconut milk
- handful of fresh cilantro leaves
- juice of 1 lime
- *OPTIONAL -1/2 t black pepper (if you have reintroduced it)*

Method:
- heat olive oil in a large soup pot over medium heat
- finely dice the onion and sauté until translucent
- add garlic, fresh and powdered ginger, turmeric, salt & dried cilantro and sauté until you smell the garlic and ginger
- add sweet potato, spinach and water (or broth) and boil until fork tender
- add shrimp and coconut milk and cook 5 more minutes
- add cilantro leaves, black pepper (if reintroduced) and lime juice
- serve with cauliflower rice or enjoy as a soup

66

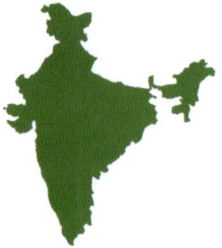

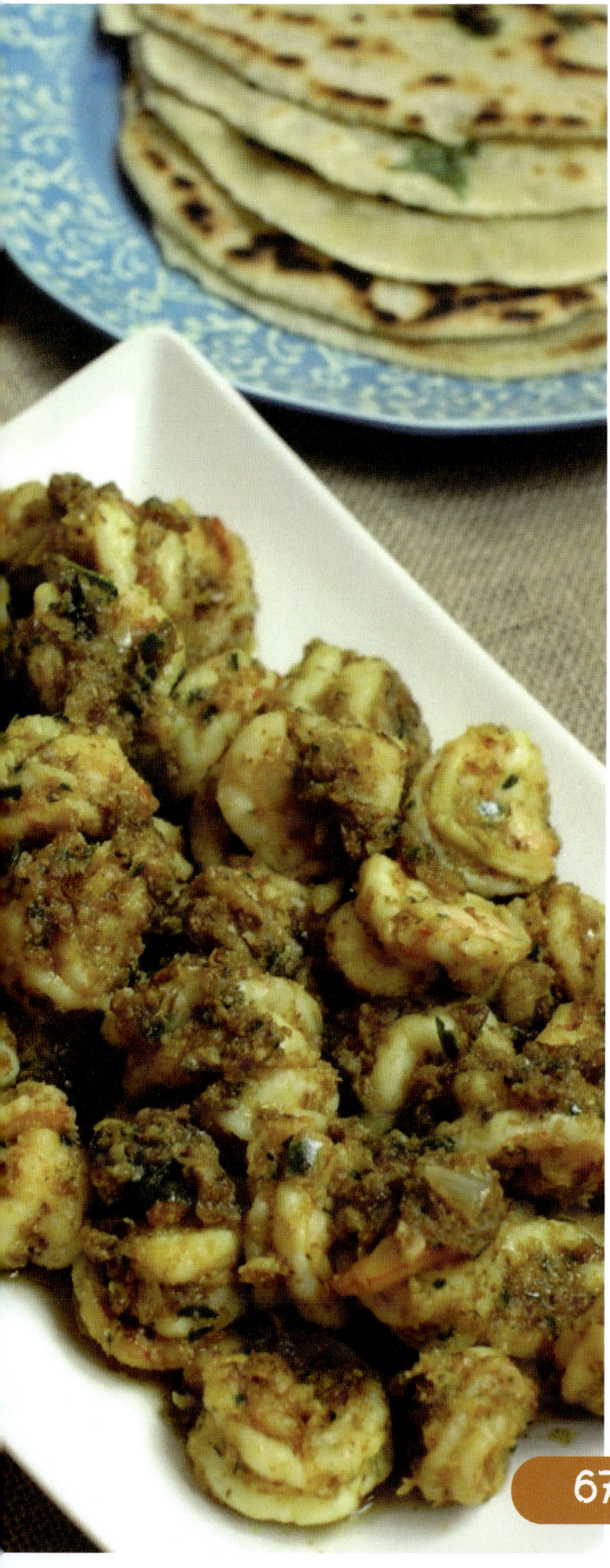

Prawn Masala

Serves: 4   Time: 45 minutes

Ingredients:

- 1 pound of shrimp/ prawns cleaned
- 1 medium red onion
- 3 cloves of garlic
- 1/2 TBSP ginger powder
- 1/2 tsp turmeric powder
- 1/2 tsp sea salt
- 1/8 tsp mace powder
- 25 curry leaves (divided)
- 2 TBSP shredded coconut
- 4 TBSP olive oil

Method:

- use a food processor to make a masala paste of the onion, garlic, ginger, turmeric, mace, salt, 20 curry leaves and 2 TBSP oil
- rinse the shrimp well and place in a bowl and coat the shrimp with the paste and allow to marinate for 10-20 minutes
- heat 2 TBSP olive oil in a large skillet over a high heat and add 5 curry leaves - allow them to cook for 1 minute
- add shredded coconut and fry for another minute
- then add shrimp and masala paste and stir fry for 3-4 minutes
- turn heat down to low and add 1/4 cup water and allow to cook for another 4 minutes until shrimp are cooked through
- serve with garlic cilantro roti

These are also fun to serve as 'tacos' in a roti with some mango chutney.

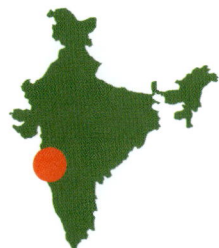

67

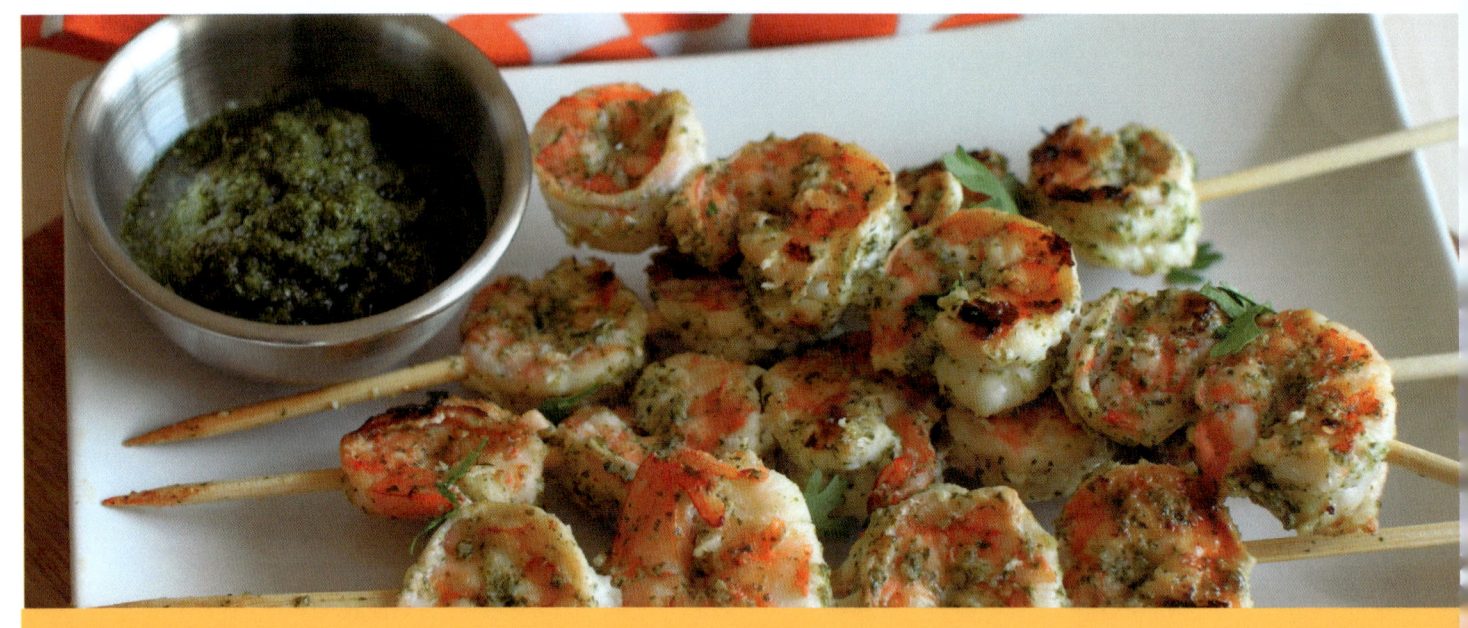

Coriander Prawn Skewers

Serves: 3   Time: 30 minutes

Ingredients:
- 1/2 TBSP olive oil
- 1 pound of shrimp
- 1 recipe of 'coriander chutney' from pg. 31
- wooden skewers

Method:
- wash the shrimp well & pat dry
- place shrimp and 1/2 recipe of coriander chutney in a large zip-top bag
- rub the chutney well over all of the shrimp and place shrimp in fridge for 20 minutes
- place wooden skewers in a baking dish and soak in water for at least 10 minutes
- after shrimp have had time to marinade, place 5-6 shrimp on each skewer
- heat a grill pan over a medium heat and drizzle with olive oil
- grill skewers for 2-3 minutes on each side until shrimp are opaque
- serve with extra coriander chutney for dipping

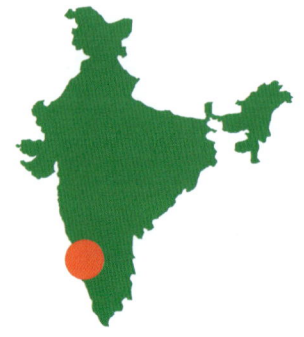

68

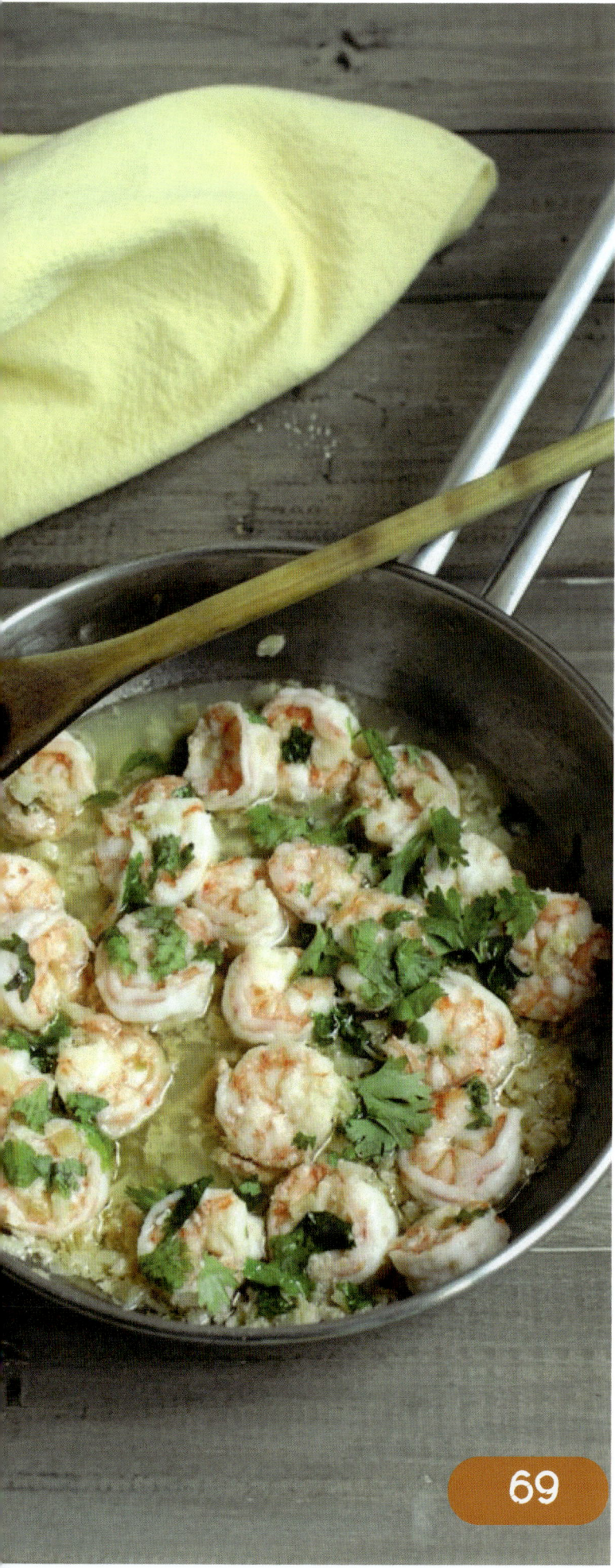

"Butter" Garlic Prawns

Serves: 2-3   Time: 14 minutes

Ingredients:
- 8 cloves of garlic
- 1 TBSP coconut oil (or ghee if reintroduced)
- 1/2 tsp dried ginger
- 1 pound of shrimp/ prawns (cleaned)
- 1/2 tsp sea salt
- 1/4 tsp turmeric
- 1 TBSP water
- 3 TBSP chopped cilantro/ coriander leaves

Method:
- finely chop or crush 8 cloves of garlic
- heat 1 TBSP coconut oil in a skillet over a medium heat
- add crushed/ chopped garlic and sauté (stirring constantly) until garlic is fragrant and getting soft, but before it starts to brown - about 4 minutes
- add ginger & turmeric and stir well to combine
- place shrimp/ prawns in the skillet
- add 1 TBSP water and stir well to combine
- reduce heat to low and cook shrimp about 4-5 minutes until all pink
- season with salt
- sprinkle coriander leaves/ cilantro over the top
- serve with Goan Mango Curry (pg. 81) and Chapatis (pg. 23) for a full meal

Reintroduction Note:
If you can eat butter or ghee, use instead of coconut oil.

Kerela Fish & Mango Curry

Serves: 4-5   Time: 50 minutes

Ingredients:
- 2 TBSP coconut oil
- 1 medium red onion
- 3 cloves garlic
- 1 TBSP dried ginger
- 1 tsp tamarind pulp
- 1 tsp dried turmeric
- 1/2 tsp mace
- 1 tsp sea salt
- 1 cup grated fresh coconut or 1 can coconut milk
- 2 cups diced pumpkin
- 1 mango - diced
- 3 cups water
- 1 pound white fish of choice (sea bream, sea bass, etc,)
- juice of 1 lime
- 1/4 cup coriander/ cilantro leaves

Method:
- dice pumpkin and mango
- heat coconut oil over a medium heat in a large saucepan
- roughly chop onion and garlic and add to pan and allow to cook for 2-3 minutes
- add ginger, tamarind, turmeric and mace and continue cooking for 1 minute
- if using fresh coconut add at this point and cook for 1-2 minutes
- add water, half the pumpkin and salt and allow to simmer for 15 minutes. Then, puree with an immersion blender
- after blending, add remaining pumpkin and mango and simmer until pumpkin is soft
- cut fish into large chunks and add to curry and simmer until fish is flaky (about 5-7 minutes)
- if using coconut milk instead of fresh coconut, add it at this point
- squeeze in lime juice and stir in coriander/ cilantro leaves and allow to simmer 3-4 minutes

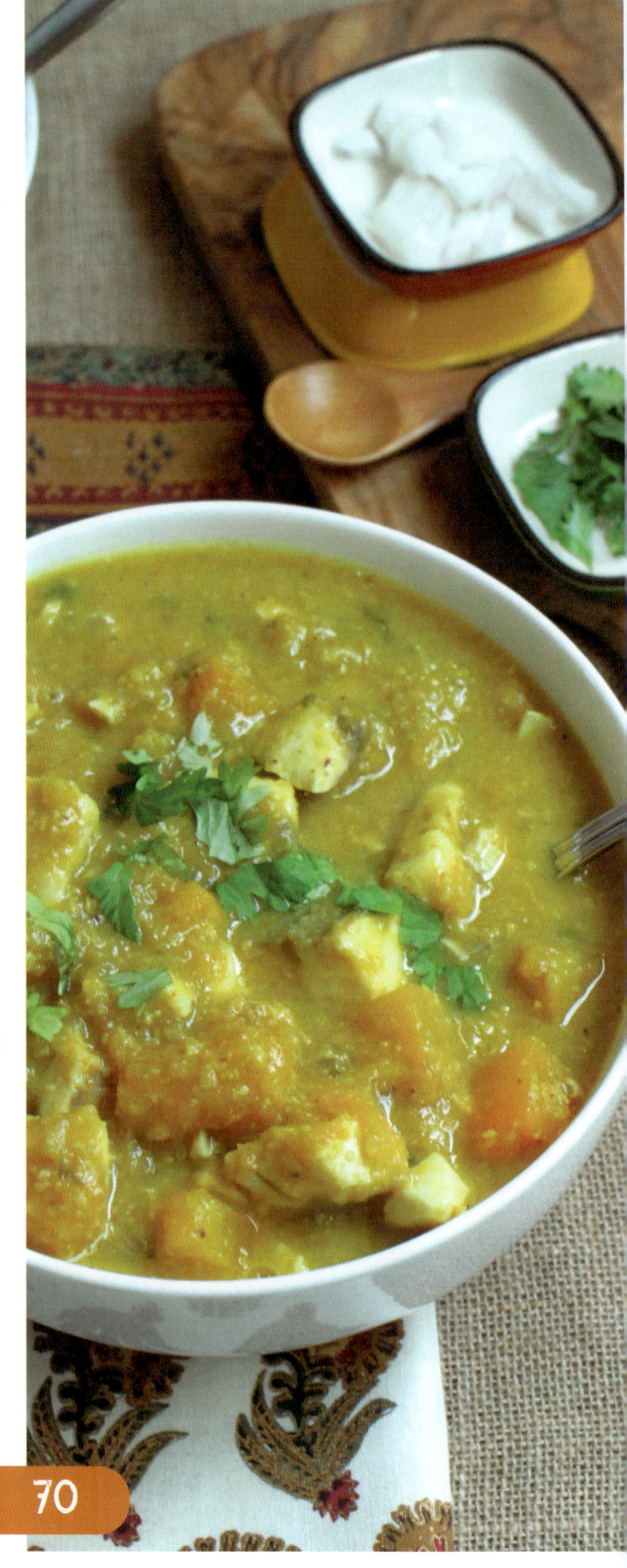

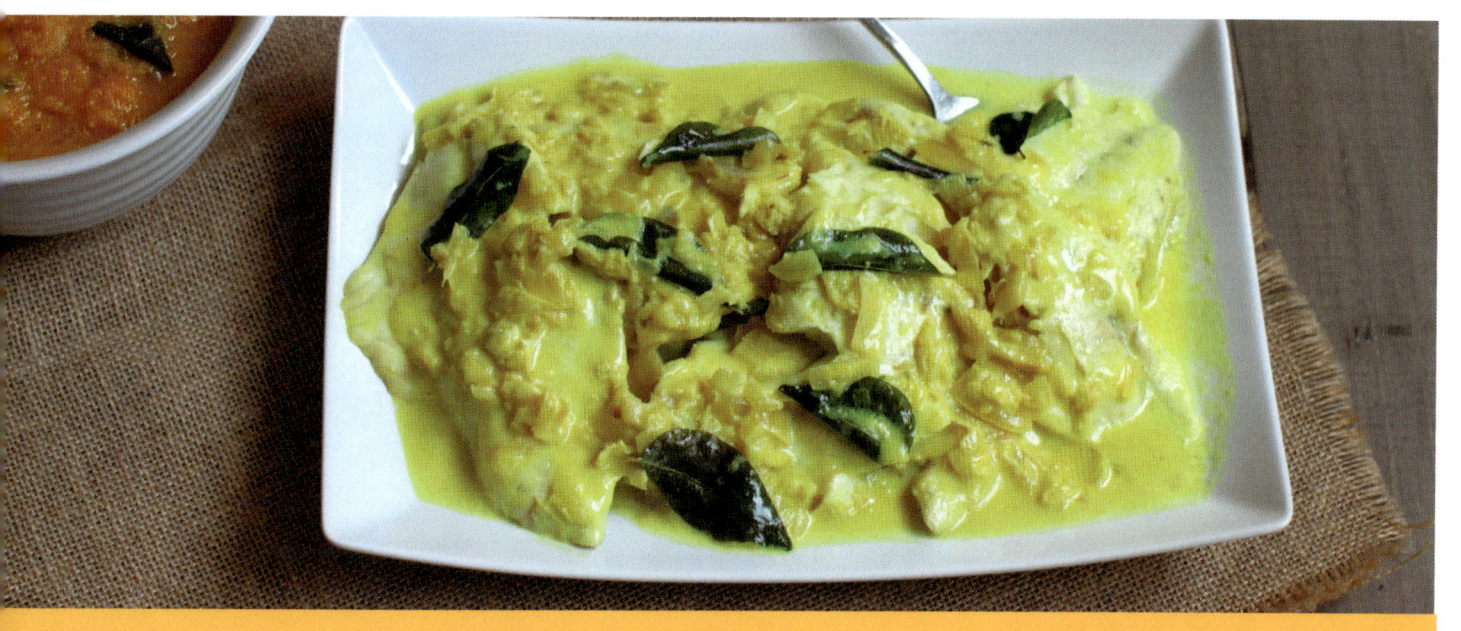

Kerala Fish Molee

Serves: 4   Time: 25 minutes

Ingredients:
- 1 medium red onion
- 2 inch piece of ginger
- 5 cloves of garlic
- 1 TBSP coconut oil
- 8 curry leaves
- 1/4 tsp turmeric powder
- 1/2 tsp sea salt
- 1 can coconut milk
- 1 pound of white fish (tilapia, pomfret, snapper) - cut into large pieces (about 3 inches)
- juice of 1 lime

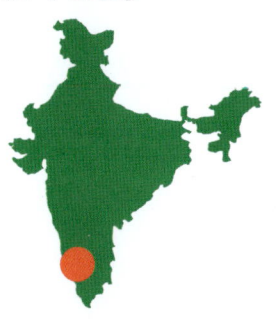

Method:
- finely dice and make a paste of onion, ginger and garlic - use a knife on your cutting board, a mortar and pestle or a food processor
- heat oil in a large skillet over medium heat
- add onion, garlic, ginger paste and curry leaves to the hot oil and fry for 2 minutes until onions are soft and starting to brown
- add turmeric and salt and fry another 30 seconds
- add coconut milk and stir well to combine and reduce heat to low - to allow sauce to simmer
- carefully place fish in coconut milk mixture
- spoon coconut milk over the fish and allow to simmer until fish flakes and is cooked through (about 5-8 minutes depending on thickness of fish)
- squeeze lime juice over fish in the last 2 minutes of cooking
- remove fish from the pan and allow sauce to reduce 5 minutes
- serve with cauliflower rice and veggies of choice

Kerala Fried Fish

Serves: 4   **Time:** 45 minutes

Ingredients:
- 3/4 tsp turmeric
- 1 TBSP ginger powder
- 1/2 TBSP garlic powder
- 1/4 tsp pink himalayan salt
- 1/2 TBSP lemon juice
- 2 TBSP water
- 8 king fish steaks (1 inch thick) - or fish of choice (NOTE: cooking times will vary with different fish) - total of 1.5 pounds of fish
- coconut oil for frying

Method:
- wash and pat dry fish pieces
- mix spices, lemon juice and water to form a paste
- rub paste on fish and allow to marinate for 30 minutes
- heat coconut oil in a large skillet over medium heat - oil should be about 1/2 inch deep
- carefully place fish in oil (oil will splatter) and allow to fry for 4-5 minutes on each side until golden brown
- allow to drain on a paper towel before serving
- serve with lemon wedges, cucumber and onion slices alongside your favorite veg dishes

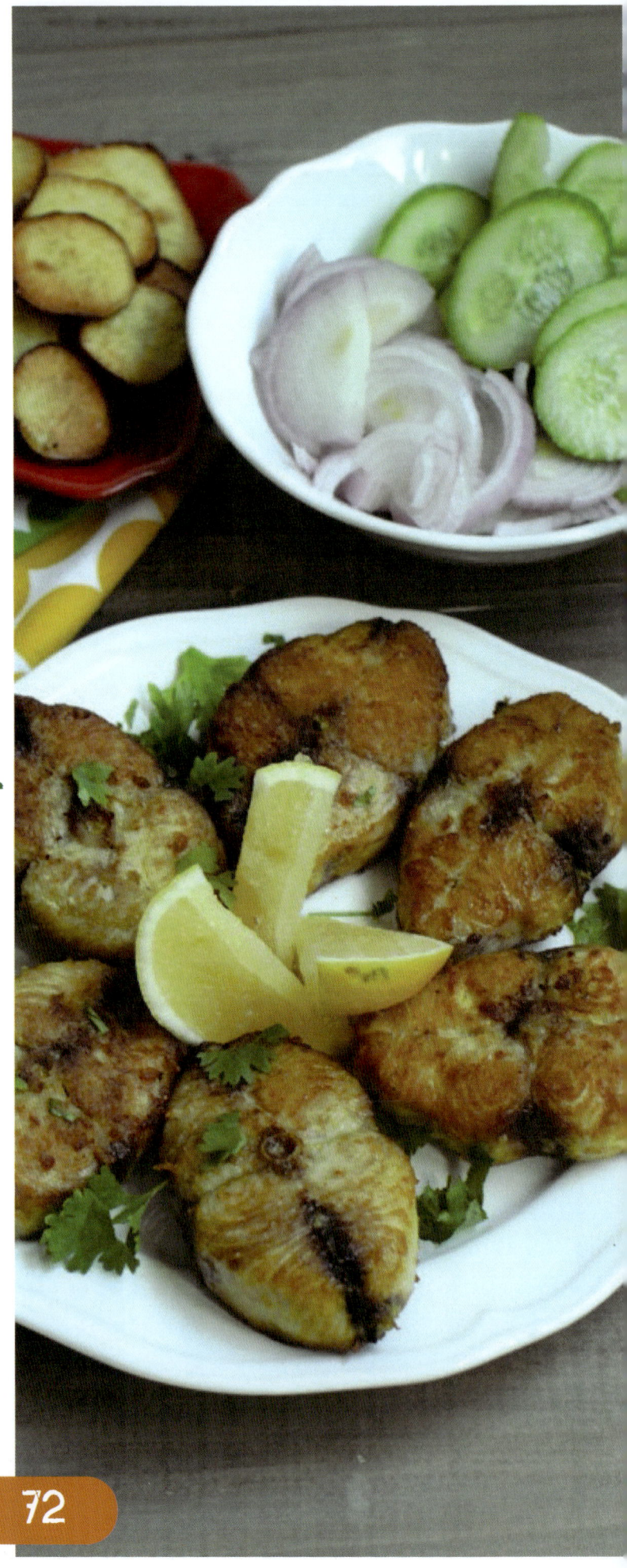

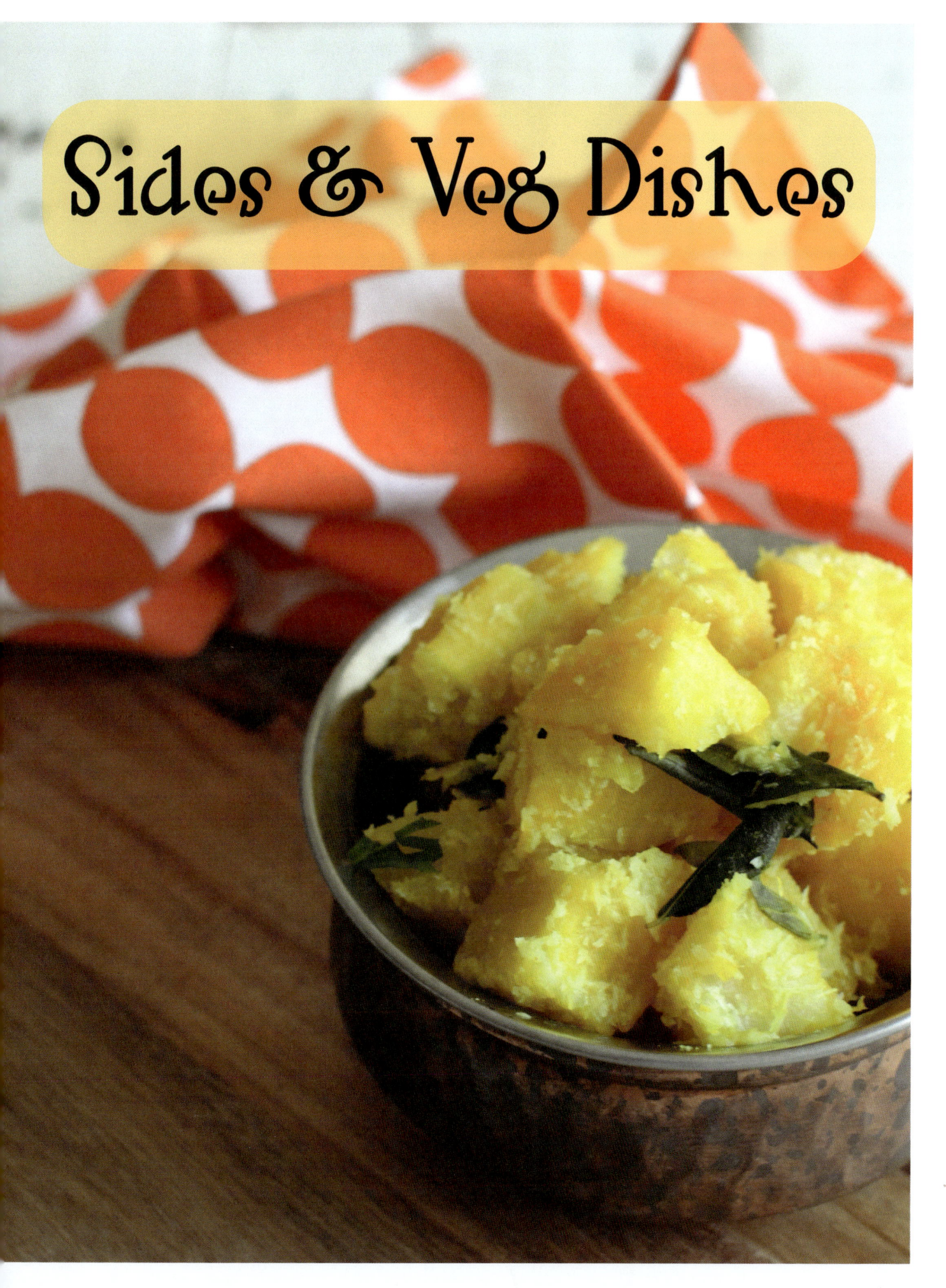

Sides & Veg Dishes

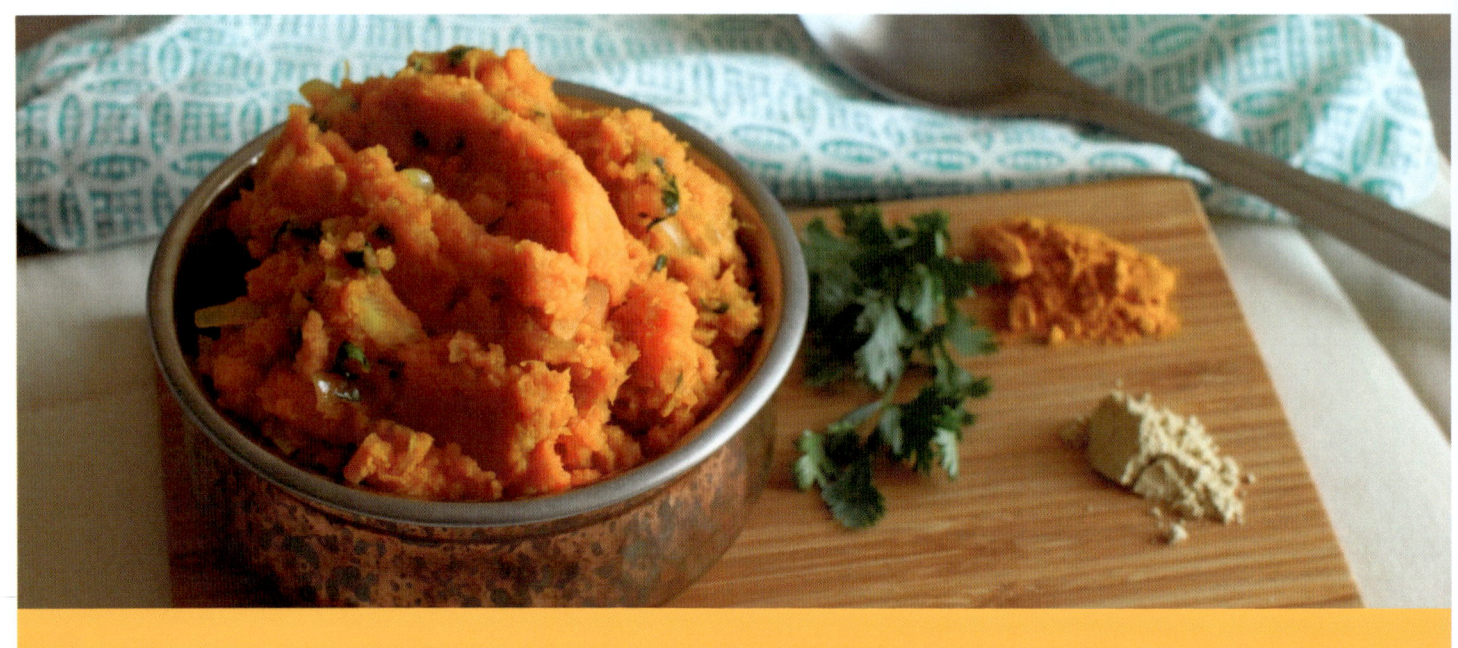

Spicy Alu Makha

Serves: 4   Time: 30 minutes

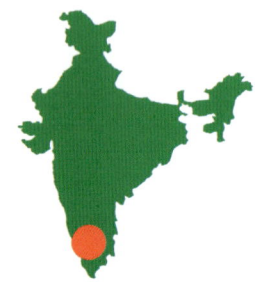

Ingredients:
- 1 pound sweet potato - peeled and chopped into 1 inch cubes
- 1 medium red onion (1/2 cup thinly sliced)
- 2 cloves garlic - crushed
- 2 TBSP olive oil
- 1 tsp pink himalayan salt
- 1/2 tsp dried turmeric
- 1/2 tsp dried ginger
- 1/3 cup chopped fresh cilantro/ coriander leaf

These sweet potatoes add an Indian flavor to all your family favorites. They're great served with meatloaf topped with the date/ tamarind chutney (pg. 34).

Method:
- peel and chop the sweet potato
- cover sweet potatoes with water in a medium saucepan, bring to a boil and cook until fork tender
- in the meantime, slice the onion and crush the garlic
- heat 1 TBSP olive oil in a small skillet and sauté the onion for 3-4 minutes, then add the garlic, salt, turmeric & ginger and continue to sauté for another 2-3 minutes until you can smell all of the spices. Remove the pan from the heat.
- once sweet potatoes are cooked, drain the water, and return to the pan add the onion mixture and 1 TBSP olive oil and mash with a potato masher.
- stir in the chopped cilantro/ coriander leaf and serve hot

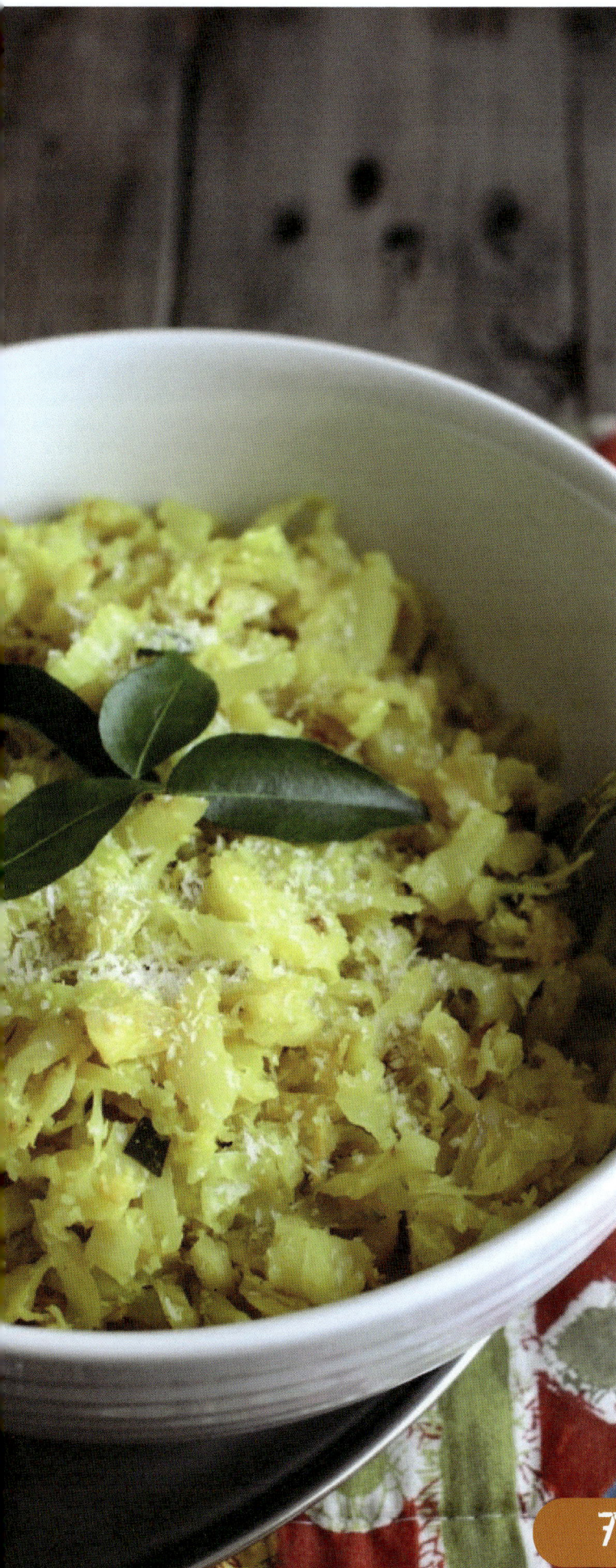

Cabbage Thoran

Serves: 4-6   Time: 40 minutes

Ingredients:
- 2 TBSP coconut oil
- 8 curry leaves
- 1 large red onion -finely diced
- 1 inch ginger -finely diced
- 2 garlic cloves -finely diced
- 8 cups shredded cabbage
- 1 tsp pink salt
- 1/2 tsp turmeric powder
- 1/3 cup shredded coconut
- 1/2 cup water

Method:
- finely dice onion, ginger and garlic and chop curry leaves into small pieces
- heat coconut oil in a large skillet over a medium heat
- add curry leaves, onion, ginger and garlic to the oil and stir fry until onions are soft and garlic and onions are starting to brown (about 4 minutes)
- add shredded cabbage, salt & turmeric and stir fry until cabbage is beginning to soften (about 8 minutes)
- add water and cook over low heat until water cooks off
- stir in coconut & serve

This is a great way to give the humble cabbage a boost!

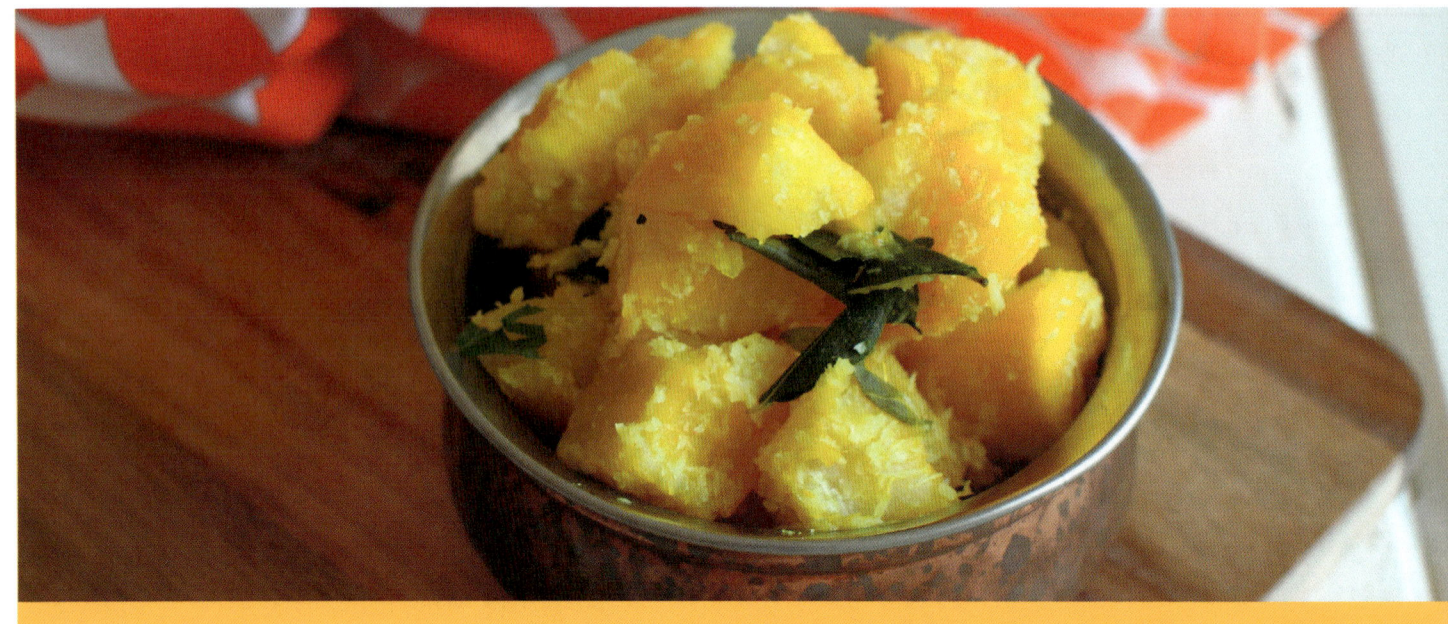

Cassava Thoran

Serves: 4   Time: 30 minutes

Ingredients:
- 1 bag of frozen cassava chunks (about a pound)
- 1 tsp pink salt (divided)
- 1/2 tsp turmeric powder
- 6 fresh curry leaves
- 1/2 tsp ground ginger
- 1/4 cup shredded coconut

Method:
- boil cassava chunks in water with 1/2 tsp pink salt, 1/2 tsp turmeric and 5-6 curry leaves until pieces are fork tender (about 25 minutes0
- if cassava pieces are large, halfway through cooking, cut into bite-sized pieces and return to the cooking water
- drain and return to the hot pan
- add 1/2 tsp pink salt, ginger and coconut powder and stir well to combine

Reintroduction Note:
If you've reintroduced mustard seeds, fry 1 tsp mustard seeds in 1 TBSP olive oil over a medium heat until they sizzle and pop and drizzle over the top of the cassava.

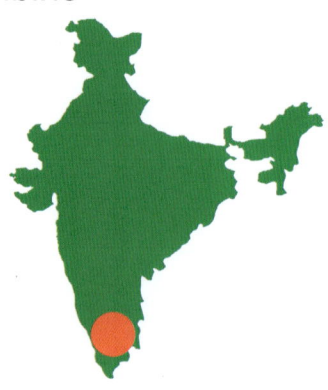

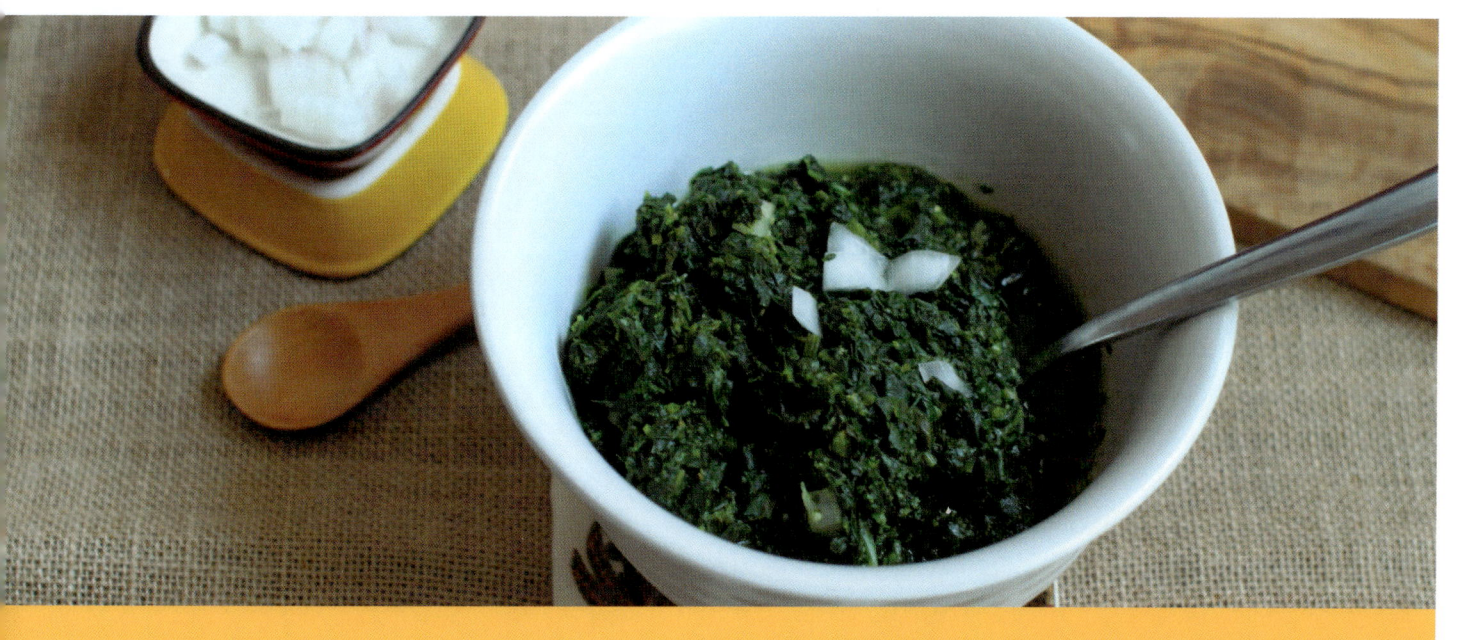

Simple Saag (Spinach)

Serves: 4   Time: 5 minutes

Ingredients:

• 2 cups of frozen spinach
• 1/4 cup chopped red onion
• 1 TBSP water
• 1 TBSP apple cider vinegar
• 1/2 TBSP dried ginger
• 1 tsp garlic powder
• 1/2 tsp turmeric
• 1/2 tsp pink himalayan salt

I love the convenience of frozen spinach. If you want to use fresh, just finely chop and cook down in a pan with a bit of water and add the same spices and seasonings.

Method:

• place frozen spinach, onion and water in a small bowl and microwave on medium for 3 minutes
• remove from microwave and stir in apple cider vinegar and spices
• serve with any of your favorite curries

If you don't want to use microwave:

• *place spinach, onion and 1/4 cup water in a saucepan over medium heat until spinach has thawed completely and heated through*
• *remove from heat and add spices and vinegar*

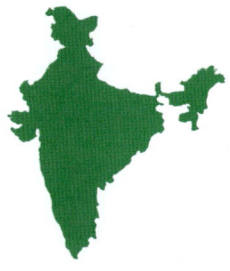

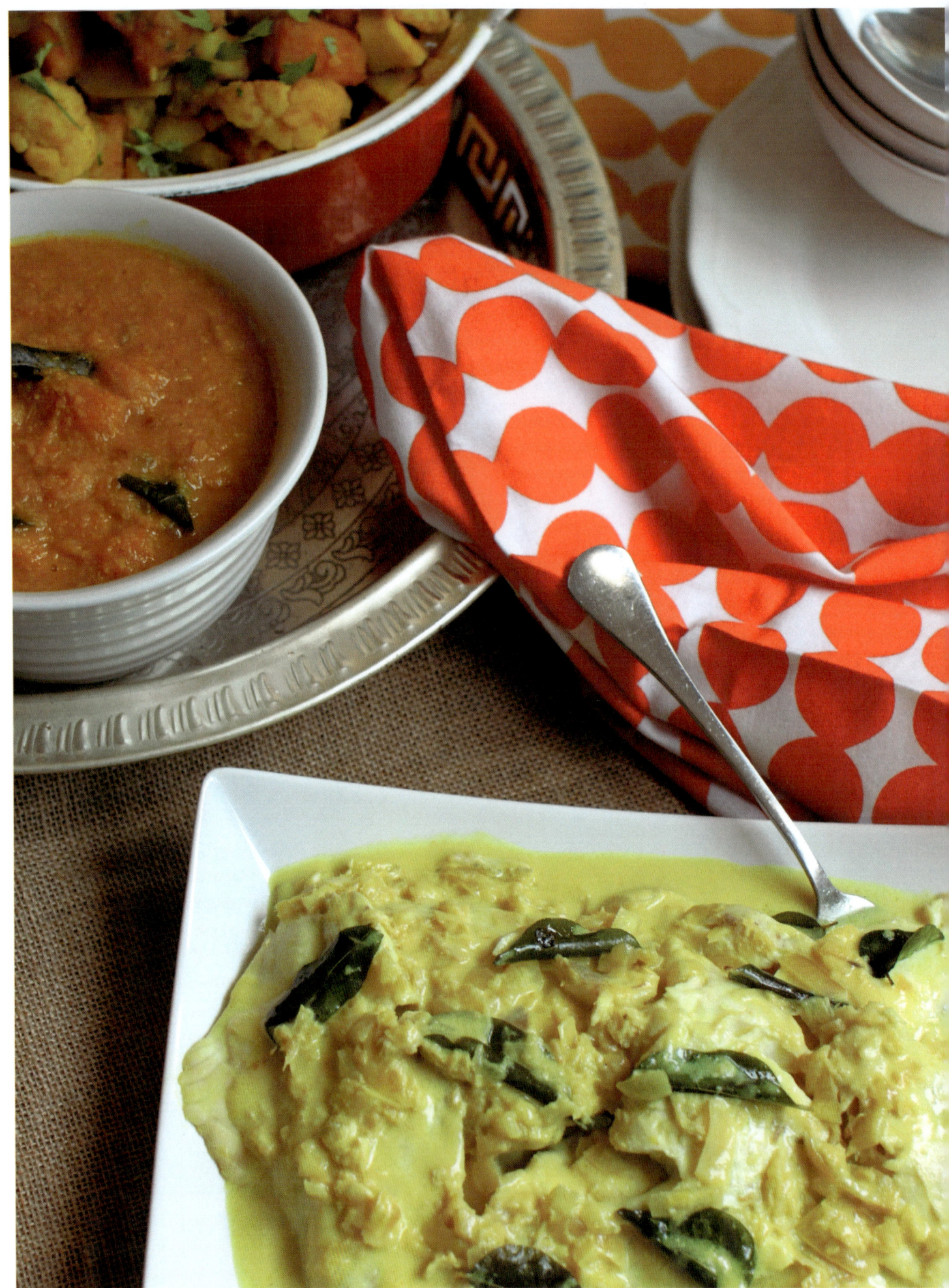

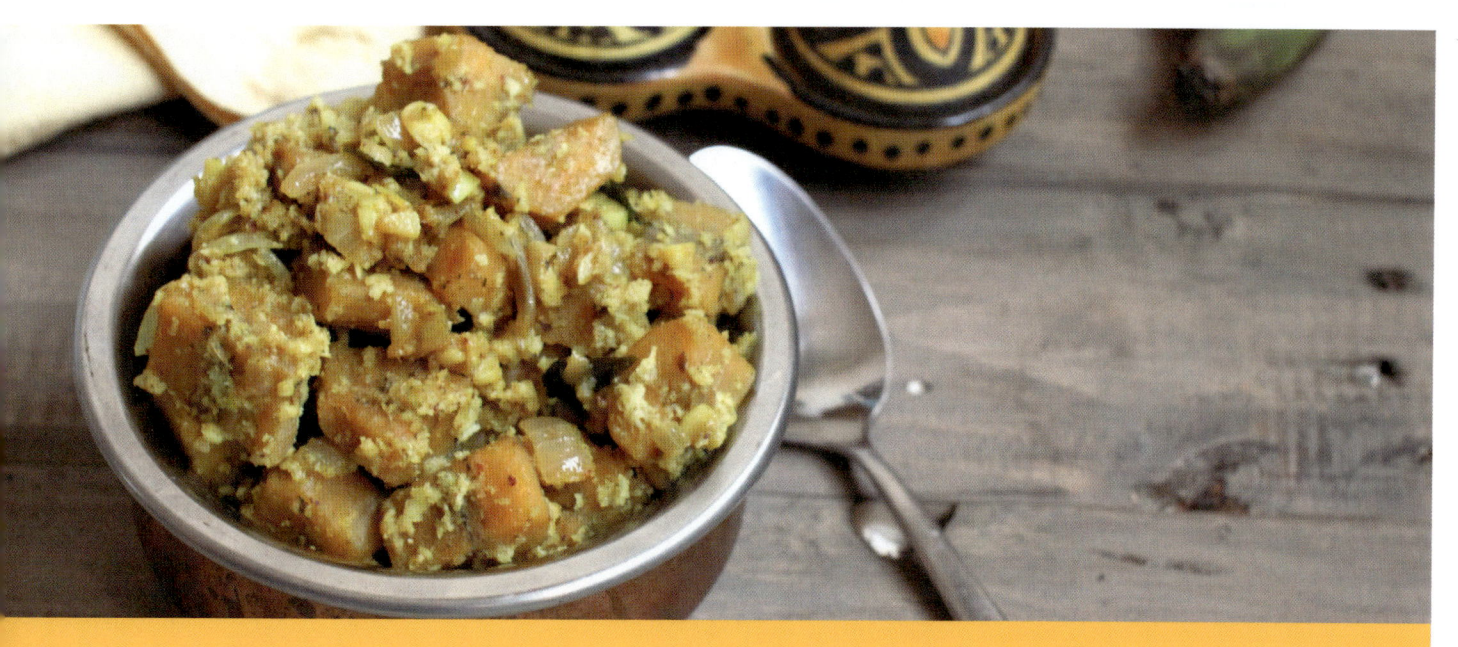

Plantains (Kacche kele ki Sabzi)

Serves: 4   Time: 40 minutes

Ingredients:

- 2 large (or 3-4 small plantains) - about 2 cups peeled and chopped
- 1 tsp tamarind paste
- 1/2 tsp sea salt (divided)
- 1 TBSP coconut oil
- 6 curry leaves
- 1 small red onion
- 5 cloves of garlic (crushed)
- 1 TBSP coconut sugar
- 1/2 TBSP dried ginger
- 1/2 tsp turmeric powder
- 2/3 cup water
- 1/4 cup grated fresh coconut

Method:

- peel and chop plantains into small cubes
- cover plantains with water and bring to a boil
- add 1 tsp tamarind paste and 1/4 tsp sea salt to the water and allow to boil for 15-20 minutes until plantains are fork tender
- finely dice the onion and crush the garlic
- in the last 5 minutes of plantain cooking, heat 1 TBSP coconut oil in a skillet over medium heat. Add the curry leaves to the hot oil and fry for 45 seconds before adding the onion and garlic. Allow curry leaves, onion and garlic to fry for 3 minutes
- drain the plantains and add to the skillet along with coconut sugar, ginger, turmeric, water and 1/4 tsp salt
- reduce heat to low and simmer until all water is cooked off
- once water is cooked off, stir in 1/4 cup of fresh grated coconut
- serve alongside your favorite curry

79

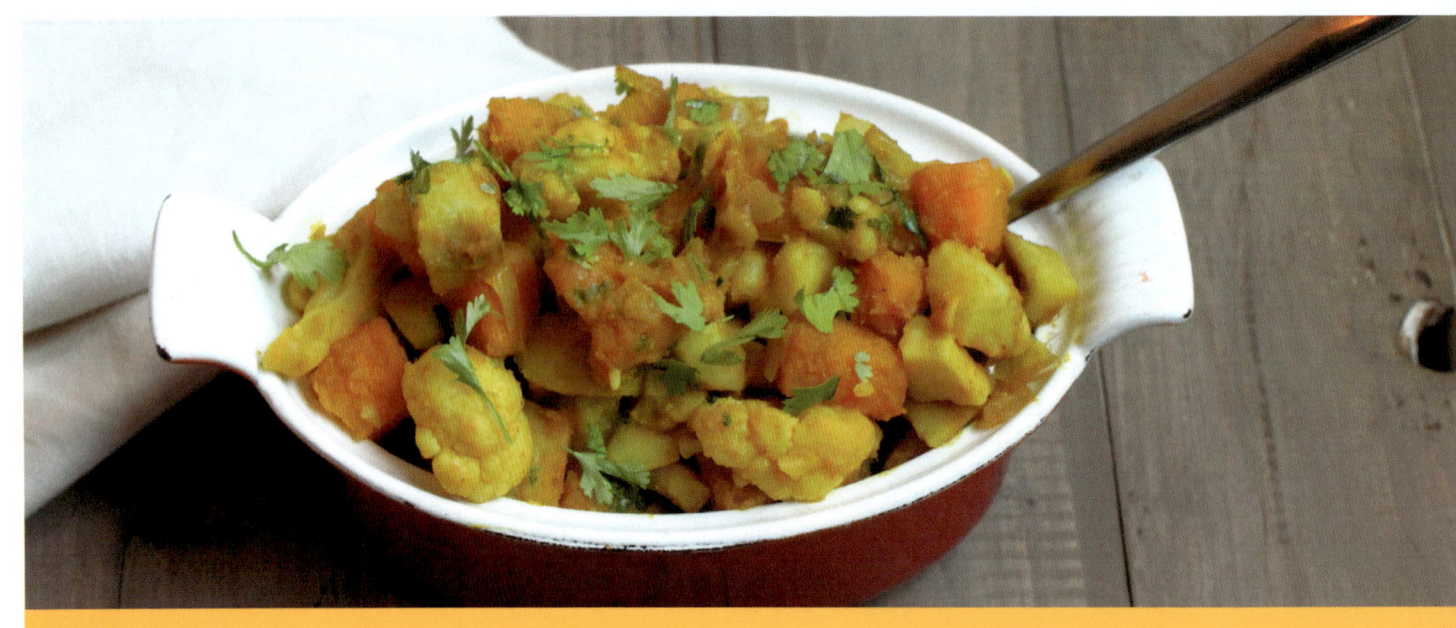

Aloo Gobi

Serves: 4-6   Time: 35 minutes

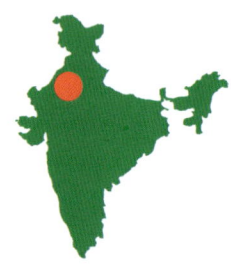

Ingredients:

- 2 cups of cubed sweet potatoes (white or orange)
- 1 medium head of cauliflower
- 1 large red onion - finely diced
- 3 cloves garlic
- 2 TBSP coconut oil
- 1 TBSP ginger powder
- 1 tsp turmeric powder
- 1/4 tsp mace
- 1/2 cup water
- 1/2 - 3/4 tsp sea salt
- 3 TBSP chopped fresh coriander/ cilantro leaves

Reintroduction Note:
If you can eat seed spices, add 1/2 tsp cumin seeds and 1/2 tsp coriander seeds with the other spices.

Method:

- wash, peel and chop sweet potatoes into bite sized pieces
- cut cauliflower into small florets
- dice onion and garlic
- heat coconut oil in a large skillet over medium to high heat
- add potatoes to the skillet and allow to fry for 4-5 minutes
- add onions, garlic and spices and fry for another 2 minutes
- add water and stir well to collect fried bits from the bottom of the skillet
- add cauliflower to the skillet, mix well, cover, reduce heat and simmer for 8 minutes until cauliflower and sweet potatoes are fork tender
- sprinkle with fresh coriander/ cilantro leaves

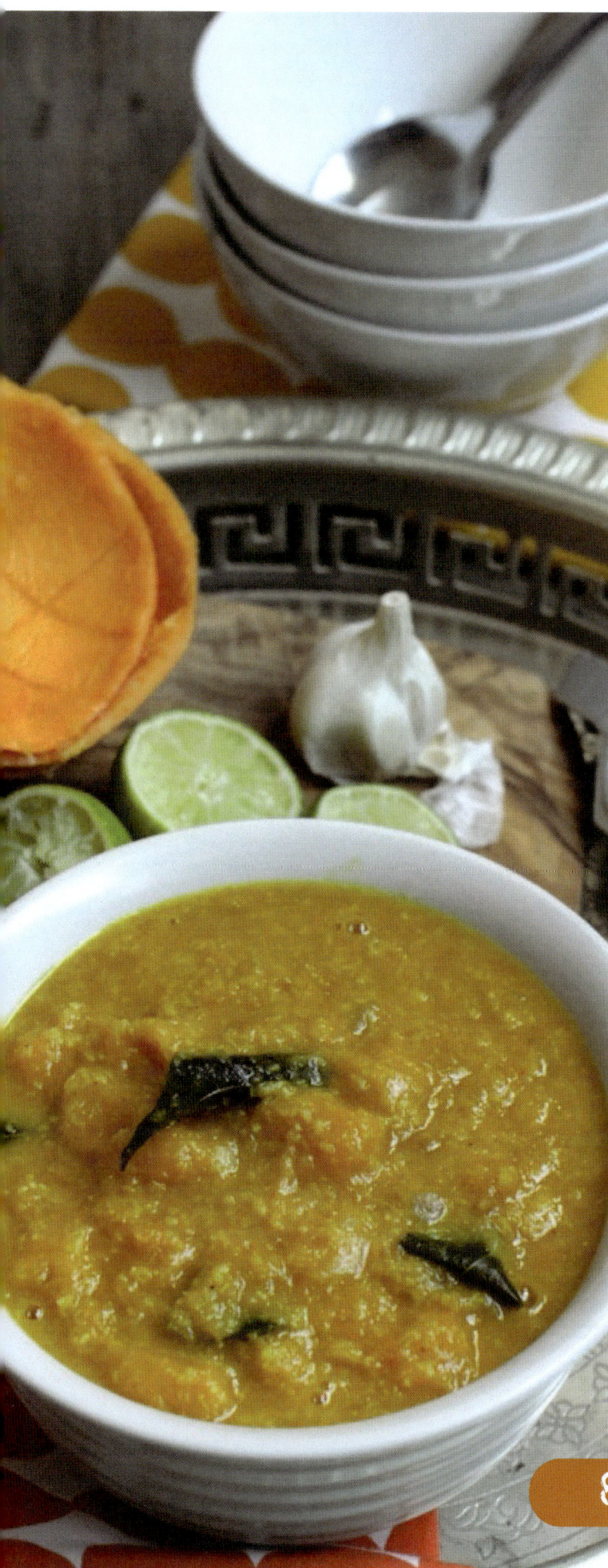

Goan Mango Curry

Serves: 4   Time: 25 minutes

Ingredients:

- 1 TBSP coconut oil
- 1/2 red onion - finely diced
- 10 curry leaves
- 1 TBSP ginger powder
- 1 tsp garlic powder
- 1/4 tsp turmeric powder
- 1/8 tsp mace
- 3/4 tsp pink himalayan salt
- 2 large (or 4 small) ripe mango - cut into bite sized pieces
- 1/4 cup grated coconut (fresh if possible)
- 2 cups water
- juice of 1 lime
- 1 TBSP coconut sugar (optional)

Method:

- prep ingredients - dice onion and chop mango
- heat coconut oil in a saucepan over a medium heat
- add onion and curry leaves and fry for 1-2 minutes
- add spices (ginger, garlic, turmeric, mace and salt) and fry until all spices are fragrant
- add mango, coconut, water and lime juice
- reduce heat and simmer for 10-12 minutes until liquid has reduced and mango has cooked down
- taste and add coconut sugar last (to taste) - should be sweet, sour and spicy all at the same time. If mango is ripe, no need to add sugar.

Bhindi do Pyaza (okra & onions)

Serves: 4   Time: 25 minutes

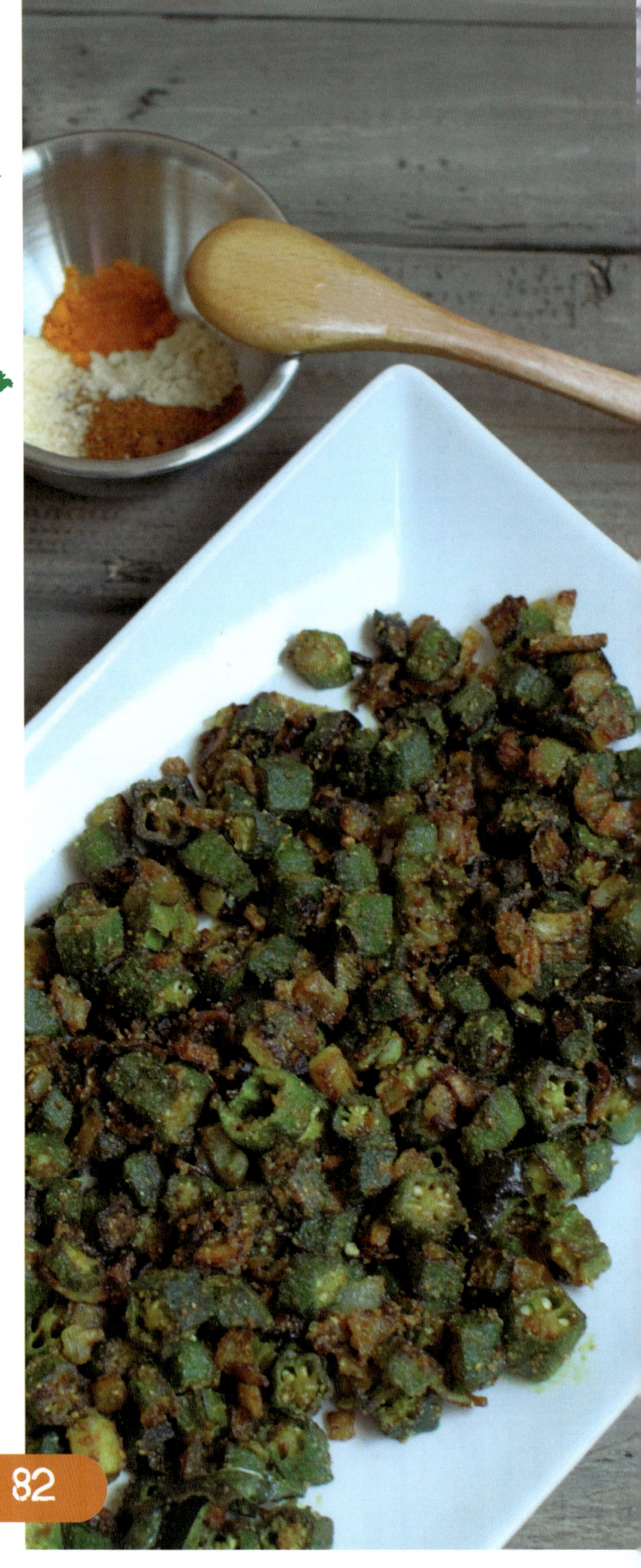

Ingredients:
- 2 TBSP coconut oil
- 3-5 curry leaves
- 1 pound of okra
- 1 large red onion
- 1/2 tsp turmeric powder
- 1/8 tsp mace
- 1/8 tsp cinnamon
- 1/4 tsp pink himalayan salt
- 1 tsp garlic powder
- 2 tsp ginger

Method:
- prep okra and onions - fine dice the onion and slice okra into 1/2 inch slices discarding the top and tip
- heat coconut oil over medium heat in a large skillet
- place curry leaves in hot oil and allow to sizzle
- add okra and cook for 4 minutes
- add onions and cook an additional 4-5 minutes (until onions start to brown)
- add all spices and cook until the raw scent of the spices cooks off (about 2 minutes)
- serve alongside any of your favorite curries or enjoy with 2-3 other vegetarian dishes and a roti for a full veg dinner

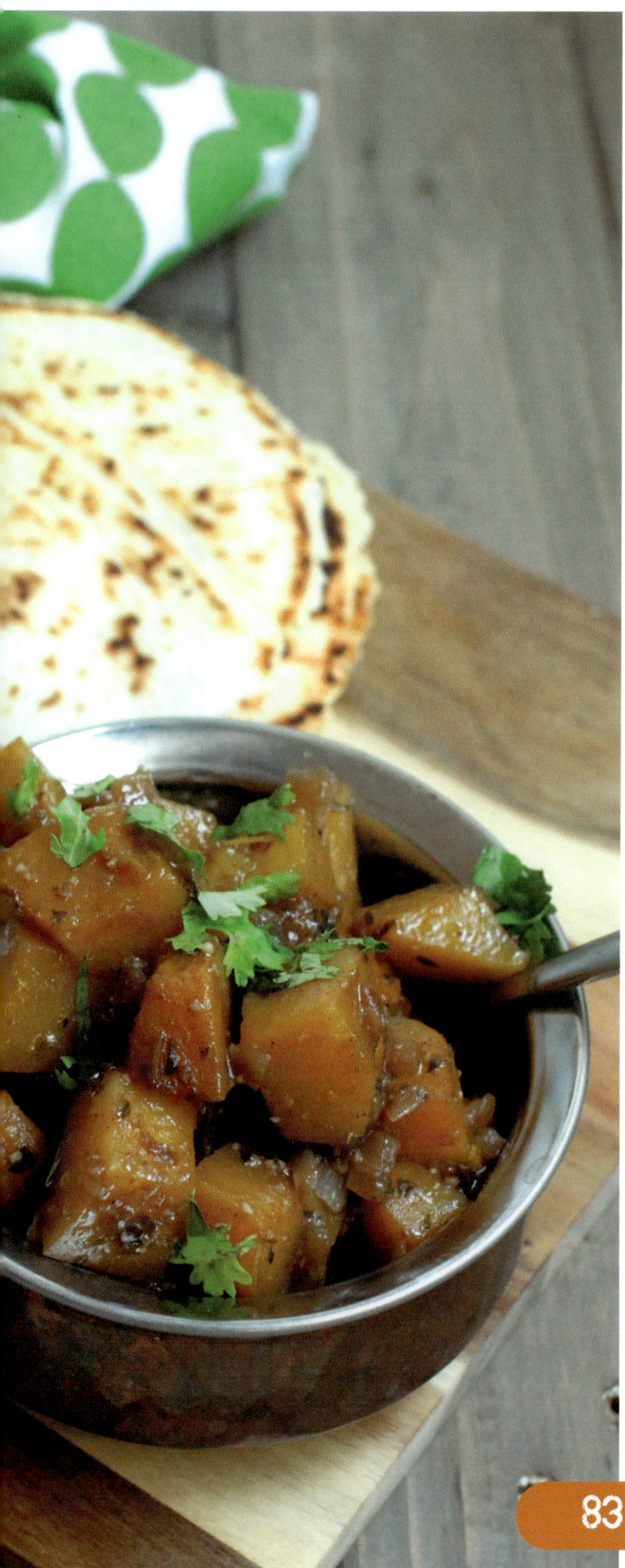

Kaddu Ki Sabzi (Pumpkin Curry)

Serves: 4 Time: 20 minutes

Ingredients:
- 1 TBSP olive oil
- 1 small red onion
- 3 cups of cubed pumpkin (or butternut)
- 1/4 tsp turmeric
- 1/8 tsp mace
- 1 tsp sea salt
- 1 tsp amchur powder
- 1 tsp garlic granules
- 1 tsp fenugreek leaves
- 1/2 tsp ginger powder
- 1 TBSP coconut sugar
- 1/4 cup water
- cilantro for garnish

Method:
- finely dice the onion
- peel and cube the pumpkin
- heat olive oil in a saucepan over a medium heat
- add onions and cook 4 minutes until starting to brown
- add spices and cook for 30 seconds before adding pumpkin and water and tossing together
- reduce to low, put a lid on the put and simmer/ steam the pumpkin until fork tender about 10-12 minutes
- garnish with cilantro leaves

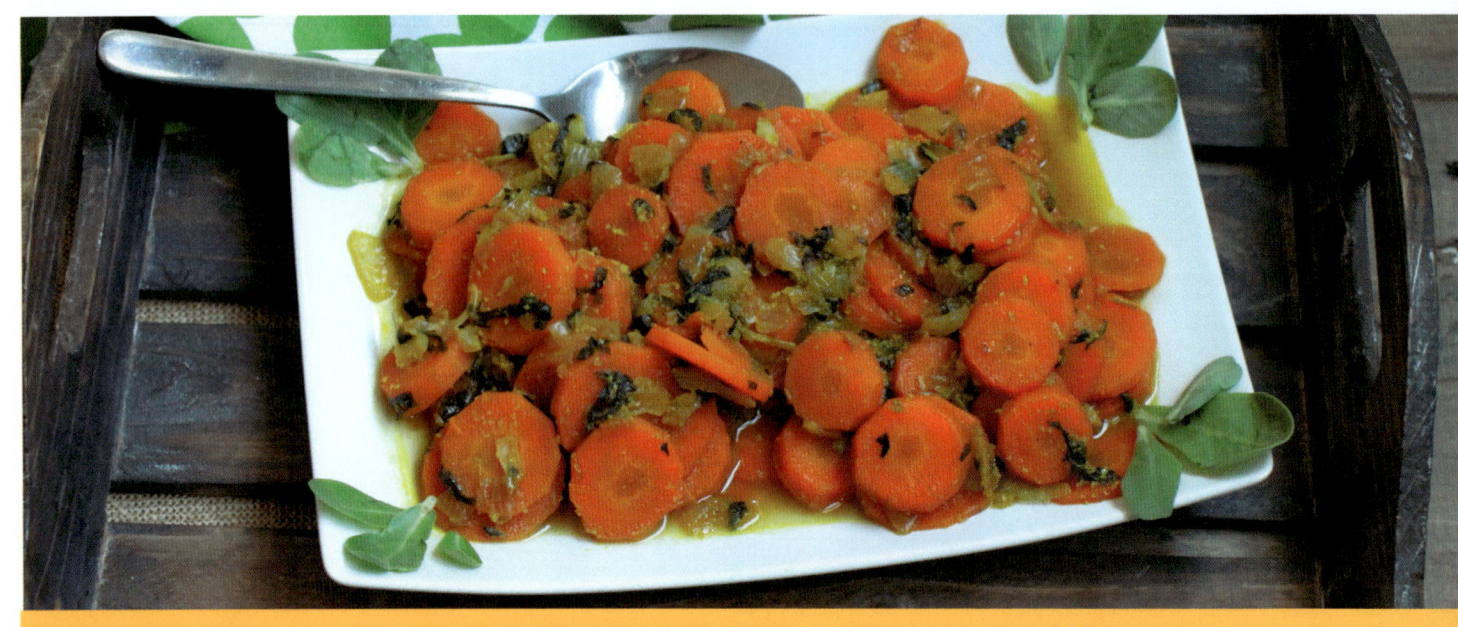

Gajar Methi Sabzi

Serves: 4   Time: 25 minutes

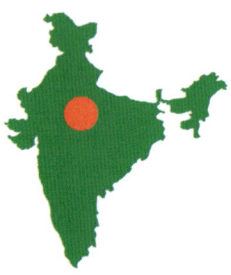

Ingredients:

- 1 small red onion - finely diced
- 1 inch piece of ginger - grated or finely diced
- 1 tsp coconut oil
- 1 tsp garlic powder
- 1/4 tsp turmeric
- 1/2 tsp coconut sugar
- 1/4 tsp sea salt
- 2 cups of sliced carrots (about 3 large carrots)
- 1 cup chopped fenugreek leaves (one large bunch)
- 1/3 - 1/2 cup water

Method:

- finely dice onion and ginger
- heat oil in a saucepan over medium heat
- allow onions to sauté 4-5 minutes (until just before browning)
- add ginger and cook another minute
- add other spices and coconut sugar and stir to combine
- add carrots, fenugreek leaves and water
- reduce heat to low, cover and allow to simmer for 8 minutes
- remove lid and cook a few more minutes until most of the water has cooked off
- serve alongside your favorite curry - especially good with lamb rogan josh

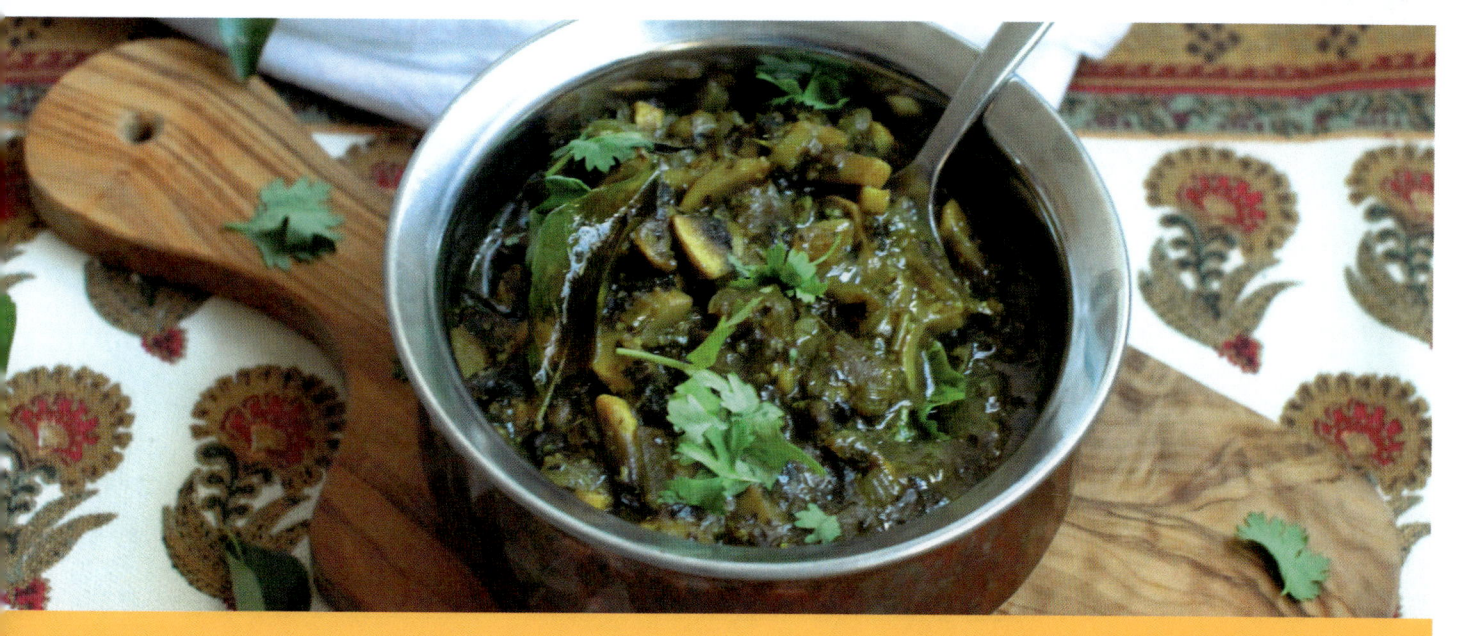

Chettinad Mushroom Masala

Serves: 4   Time: 25 minutes

Ingredients:
- 1 medium red onion
- 1 inch ginger - finely minced
- 1 TBSP coconut oil
- 8-10 curry leaves
- 2 tsp garlic powder
- 1/4 tsp turmeric powder
- 1 tsp ginger powder
- 1/8 tsp mace
- 1/4 tsp amchur powder
- 1 TBSP dried fenugreek
- 1/2 cup water
- 3 cups chopped mushrooms
- 1/4 tsp sea salt
- 2 TBSP cilantro leaves

Method:
- finely dice a small onion and a 1 inch piece of ginger
- heat oil in a saucepan over medium heat
- sauté onion for 4 minutes
- chop mushrooms while onions cook
- add ginger and curry leaves and continue cooking for 2 minutes
- add all spices and stir to combine
- add mushrooms and water - reduce heat to low - simmer for 5-6 minutes
- add salt and cilantro
- serve as a side dish to your favorite curry or as a key part of Delhi Style Aloo Tikki Chaat (pg. 45)

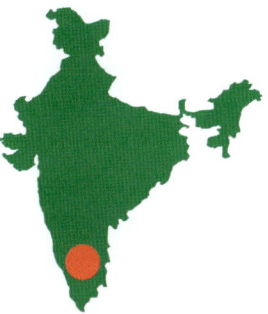

Yellow Dal (Legume - free)

Serves: 4   Time: 25 minutes

Ingredients:
- 1 TBSP olive oil
- 1 large red onion
- 1 carrot - finely diced
- 4 cloves garlic
- 8 curry leaves
- 1 tsp turmeric
- 2 tsp ginger
- 1/8 tsp mace
- 1/8 tsp cinnamon
- 1/2 tsp pink himalayan salt
- 1 cup shredded coconut
- 4 cups water

Method:
- heat olive oil in a saucepan over medium heat
- finely dice the onion and carrot and add to hot oil
- allow veggies to sauté 3-4 minutes
- dice garlic and add it to the pot... allow to sauté for 2 more minutes
- add curry leaves, spices and coconut and fry for 2 minutes
- add water, reduce heat, allow to simmer for 15-20 minutes until carrots are tender
- use an immersion blend to blend - don't completely puree - leave a few chunks of onion

NOTE: *Eat as a side dish with roti along with biryani or other curries. OR... use as a curry sauce by adding some veggies and fish.*

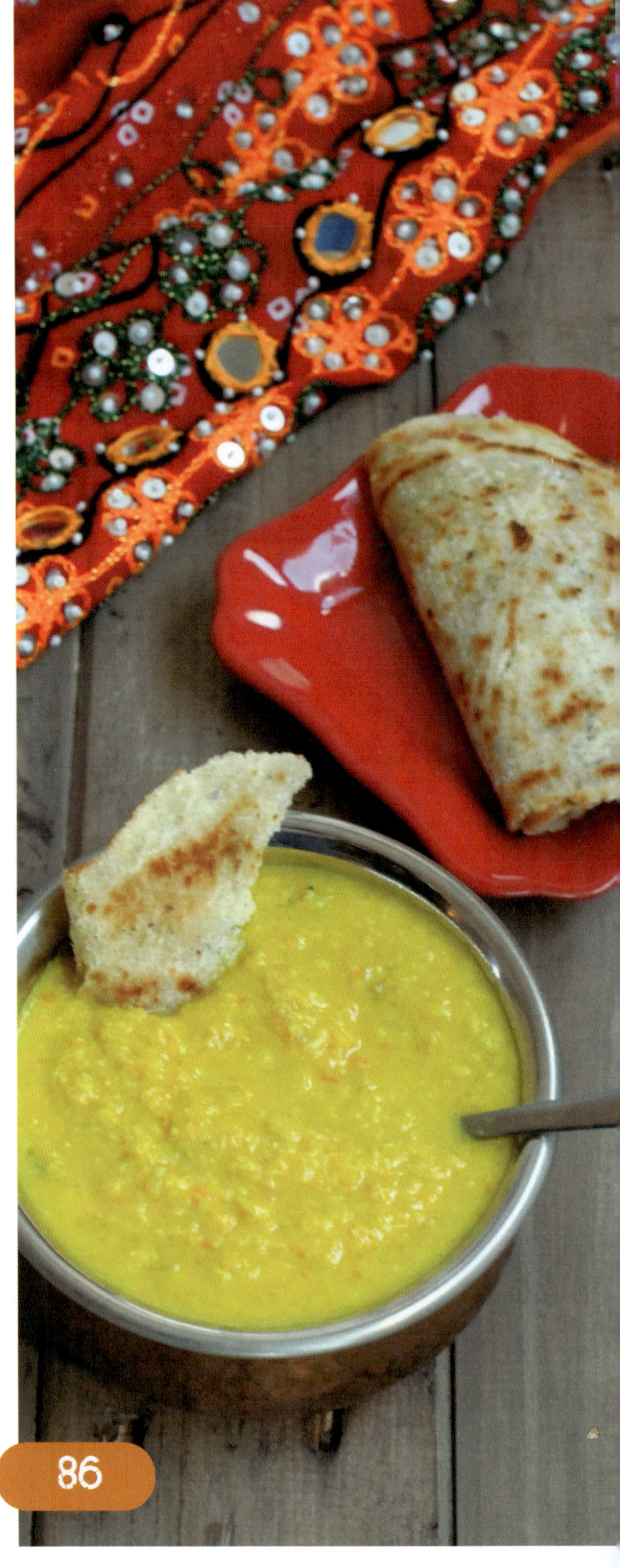

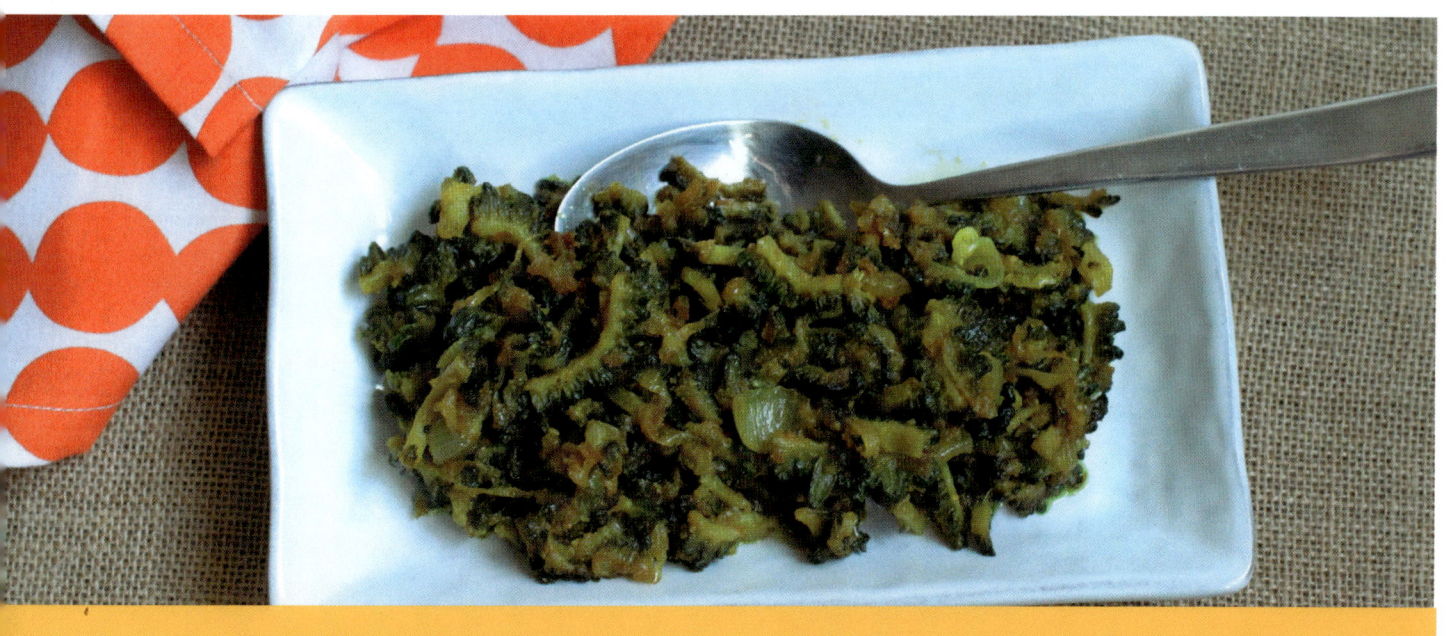

Spiced Bitter Gourd

Serves: 4   Time: 75 minutes

Ingredients:

- 2 medium bitter gourds
- 1 tsp sea salt (divided)
- 2 TBSP olive oil
- 1 large red onion
- 1 tsp garlic powder
- 1 TBSP ginger powder
- 1/4 tsp mace
- 1/4 tsp turmeric
- 1 TBSP coconut sugar

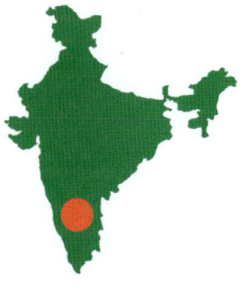

Method:

- cut the bitter gourd in half lengthwise and scoop out the seeds
- thinly slice (as thin as you can) the bitter gourd and place in a bowl
- sprinkle with 1/2 tsp sea salt and massage with your hands for a few minutes- set aside for 45 minutes
- rinse bitter gourd
- in a small skillet, heat olive oil and add onions, rinsed bitter gourd and spices (all but salt)
- allow to stir fry on low/ medium heat for 25 minutes - stirring occasionally
- add 1/2 tsp salt and coconut sugar and cook another 5 minutes
- serve along with other favorite veg dishes

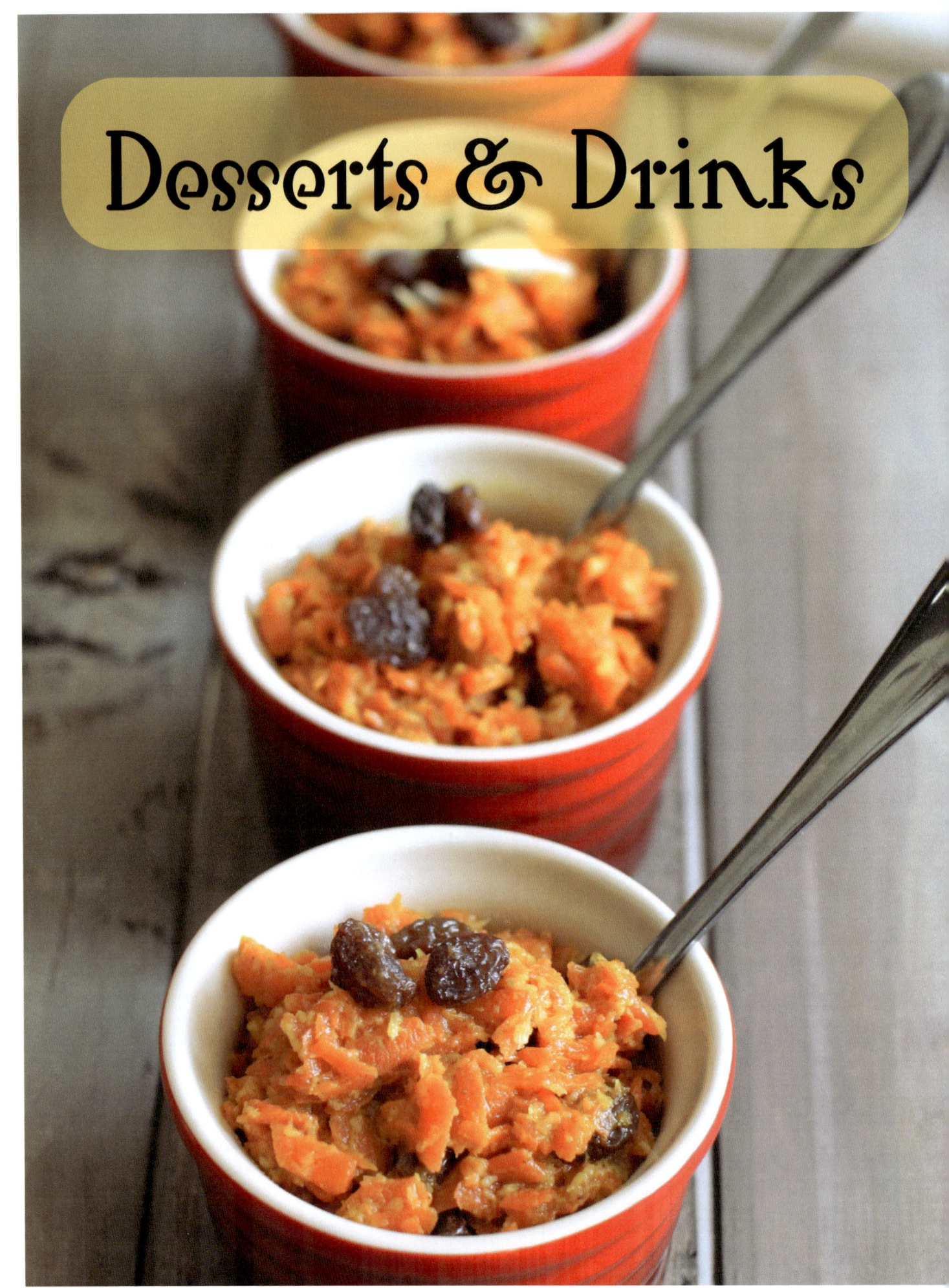

Desserts & Drinks

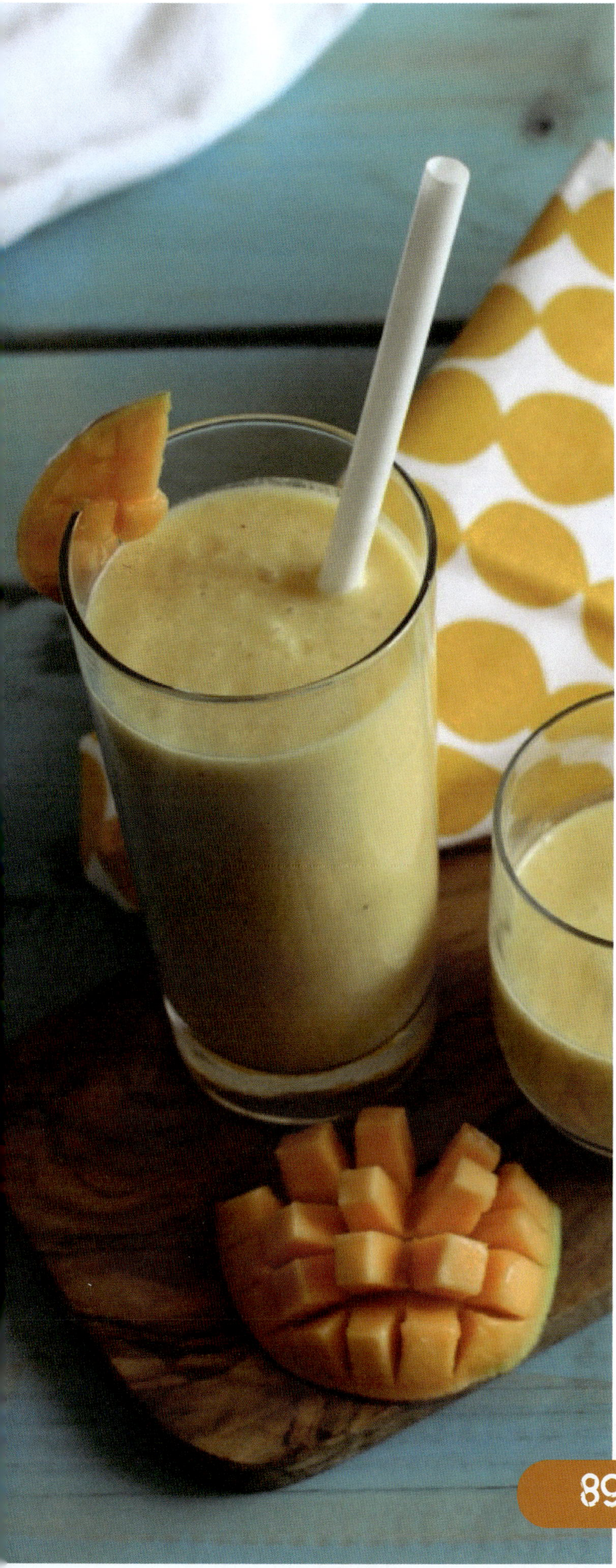

Mango Lassi

Serves: 2-3   Time: 5 minutes

Ingredients:
• 2 small mangoes (or 1 1/2 large mangoes)
• 1/4 tsp dried ginger powder
• 1/8 tsp cinnamon powder
• 1/8 tsp turmeric powder
• 1 TBSP honey
• 1 1/2 cups coconut milk (one can)

Method:
• cut mango into bite sized pieces
• place all ingredients in a blender and blend until smooth
• Lassi is supposed to be both sweet and tart. If mangoes aren't sweet you may want to add a bit more honey.
• pour into glasses and enjoy

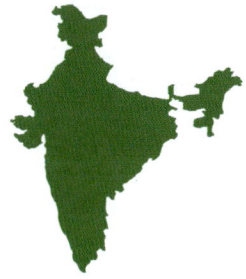

Reintroduction Note:
If you've reintroduced yogurt, or have access to coconut yogurt, replace 1/4 cup of coconut milk with yogurt.

Jal Jeera
(Spiced Lemonade)

Serves: 2   Time: 5 minutes

Ingredients:
- handful of cilantro leaves
- handful of mint leaves
- 1 TBSP honey
- pinch of pink himalayan salt
- 1 tsp tamarind pulp
- 1 TBSP crushed ginger
- juice of 1 lemon
- 1/4 tsp amchur powder
- 2 cups of water
- ice

Method:
- place all ingredients (except ice) in a blender and blend until smooth
- pour through a fine mesh strainer
- serve by pouring over ice
- garnish with lemon slices and mint leaves

Reintroduction Note:
If you've reintroduced seed spices, add half a tsp of roasted cumin seeds. Roasted in a dry pan over medium heat for a minute and grind in a spice grinder.

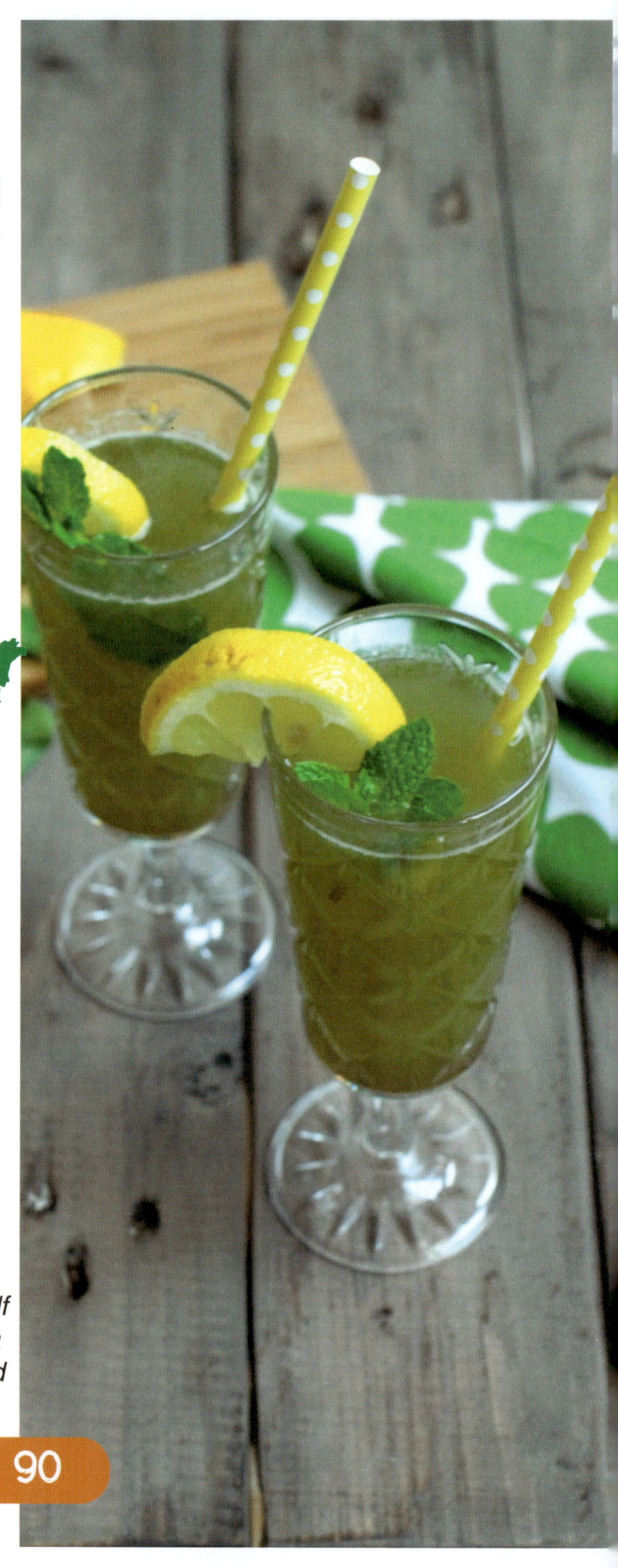

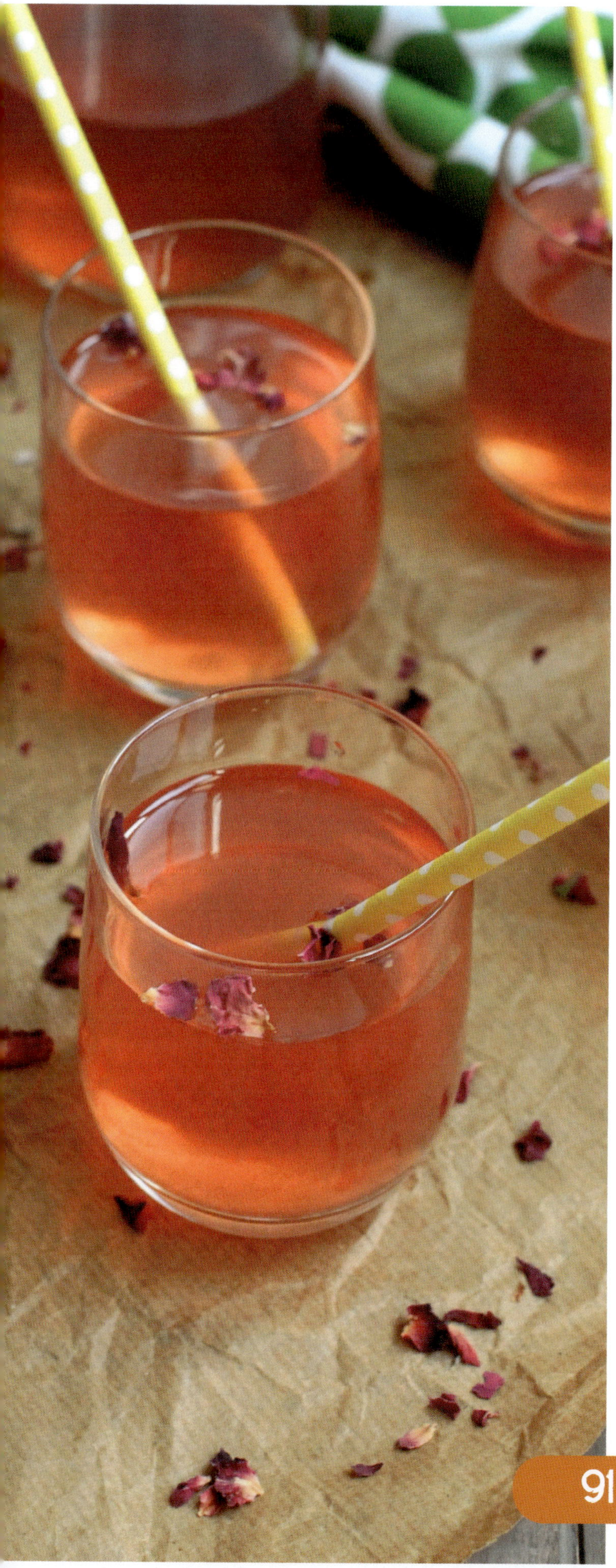

Shahi Gulab Jal
(Rose Scented Iced Tea)

Serves: 4   Time: 15 minutes

Ingredients:
- 1 cup dried rose petals
- 3 bags green tea
- 1 TBSP honey
- 2 TBSP lemon juice (about 1 lemon)
- 6 cups water (2 hot and 4 cold)
- ice for serving

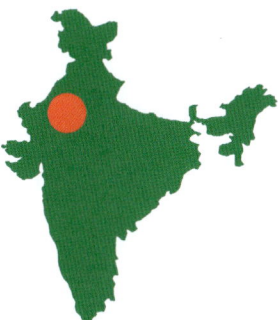

Method:
- steep rose petals in 2 cups hot water (just shy of boiling) for 10 minutes
- strain out rose petals
- add tea bags and steep an additional 3 minutes
- remove tea bags and stir in honey and then lemon juice
- top up with cold water and ice
- garnish with a few rose petals
- serve cold

This is based on a drink we were served in Jaipur and my hubby named it the royal rose drink as we felt like royalty sipping it.

Thirst Quencher
(Lemon, Ginger, Mint)

Serves: 6-8   Time: 8 minutes

Ingredients:
- 2 lemons
- 2 inch piece of ginger
- 1/2 cup of mint leaves
- 10-12 cups of water

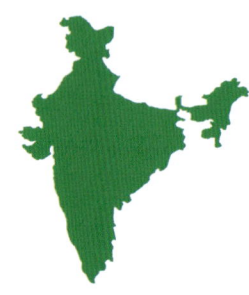

Method:
- remove peel from lemons and cut into slices or segments *(leaving the peel makes water bitter)*
- peel and thinly slice the ginger
- place lemon and ginger in a large pitcher
- heat 2 cups of water and pour over the lemon and ginger – allow to steep in hot water for 5 minutes
- remove mint leaves from stems
- fill the pitcher with cold (filtered) water
- add mint leaves and stir
- cover and refrigerate for at least 2 hours and up to 3 days
- enjoy cold
- optional – garnish with lemon slices and mint leaves

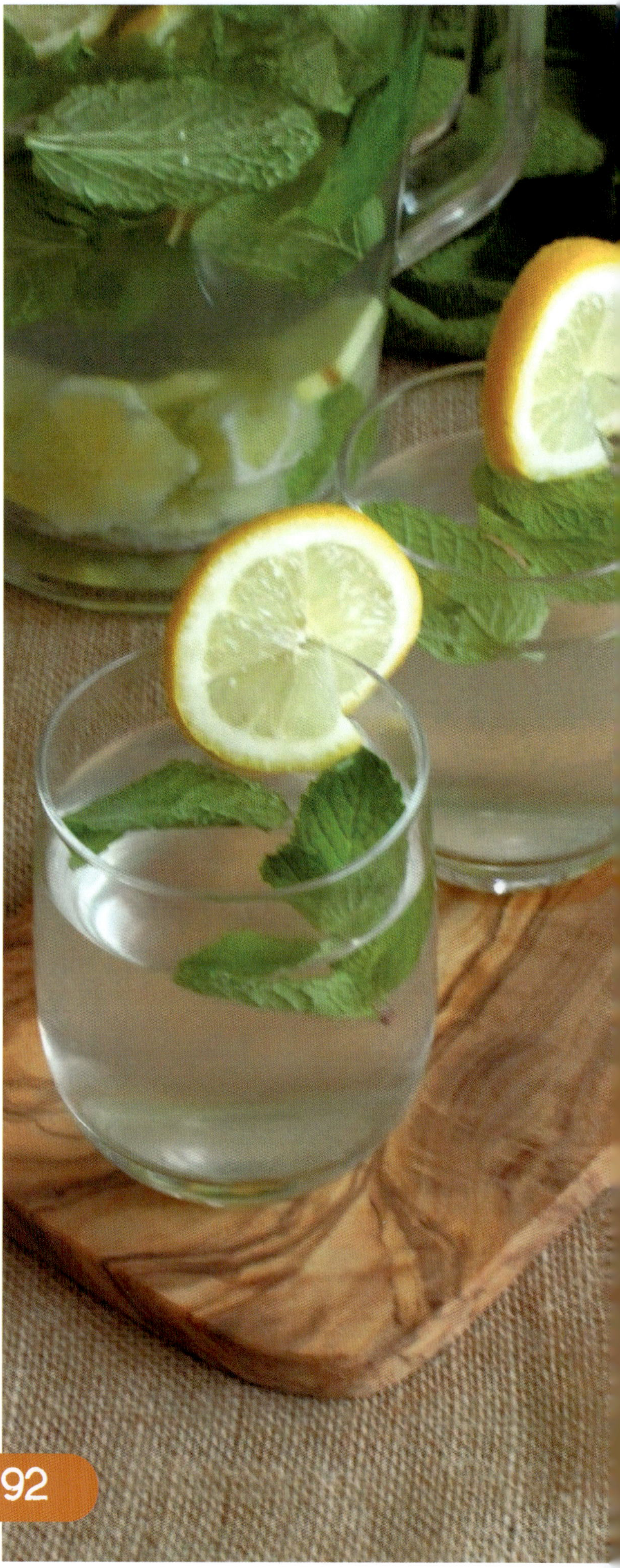

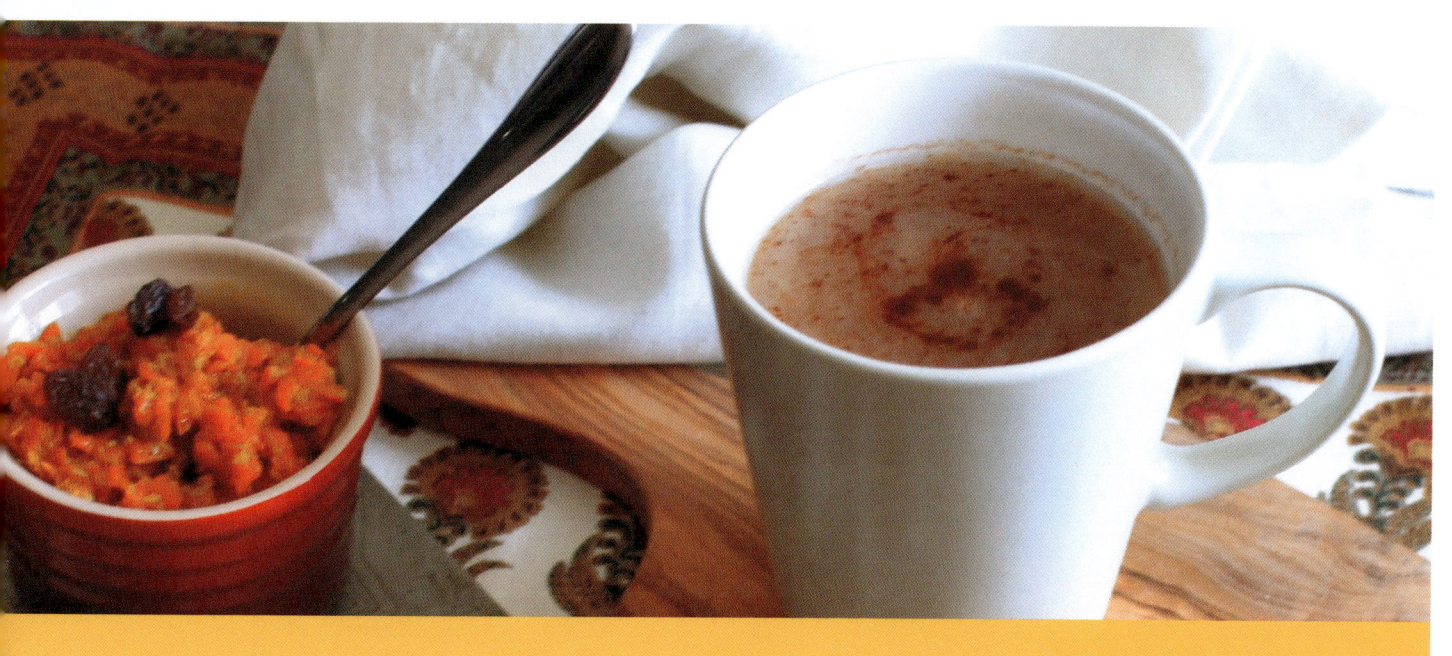

Coconut Masala Chai

Serves: 1 • Time: 5 minutes

Ingredients:
- 1 cup of tea (black, green or rooibos)
- 2 1/2 TBSP coconut milk
- 1/8 tsp mace
- 1/8 tsp cinnamon
- 1/2 tsp maple syrup

Method:
- steep a tea bag in a mug 2/3 full of boiling water (or use loose tea if you have it)
- once to your desired strength, remove tea bag and add remaining ingredients
- stir well (or blend with a milk frother for best results)
- enjoy with your favorite 'chai time' treats like carrot halwa or gulab jamun

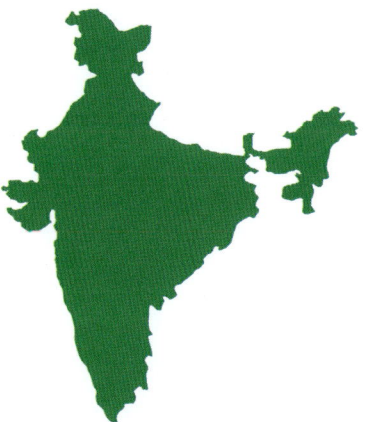

Kahwa
(Saffron Spiced Tea)

Serves: 4   **Time:** 15 minutes

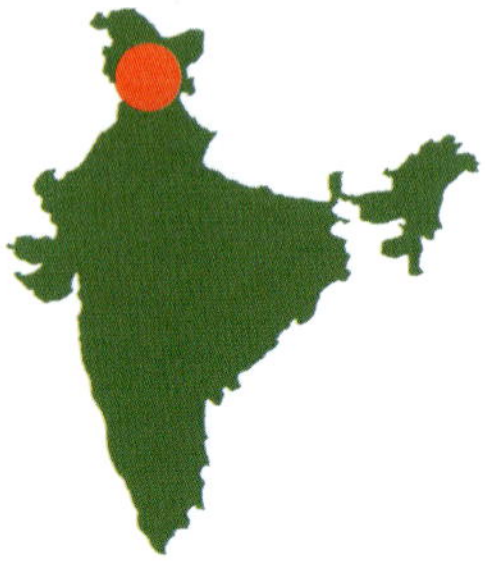

Ingredients:
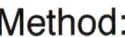
- 3 cups of water
- 1 cinnamon stick
- 1/8 tsp mace
- 2 pinches of saffron
- 2 bags green tea
- 2 tsp honey

Method:
- heat water in a saucepan and simmer cinnamon, mace and saffron for 7-8 minutes
- remove from heat and add tea bags
- allow tea to steep for 3 minutes
- remove tea bags and cinnamon stick and strain
- add honey and pour into tea cups
- garnish with 2-3 saffron strands per cup

Reintroduction Note:
If you've reintroduced cardamon, add 2 pods to the pot while simmering the saffron, cinnamon and mace. If you've reintroduced almonds or pistachios - add 1 tsp chopped nuts to each cup before pouring the tea.

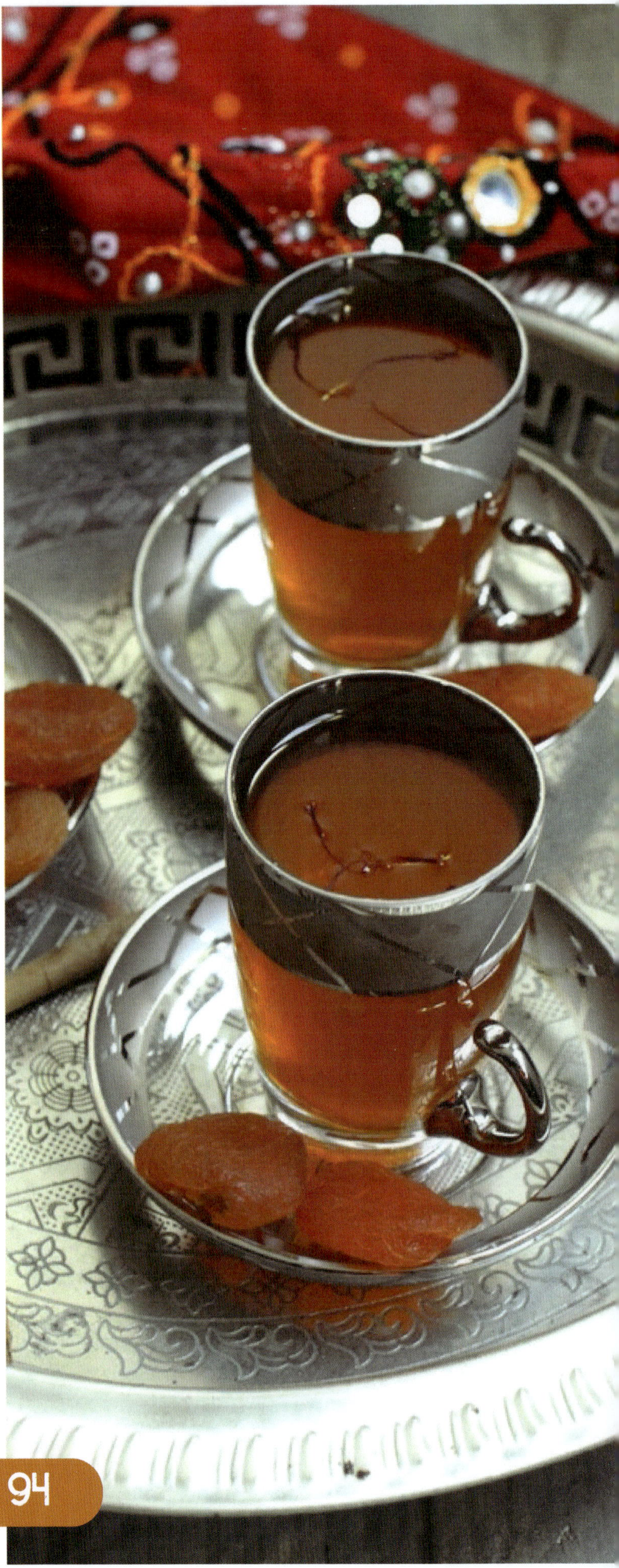

94

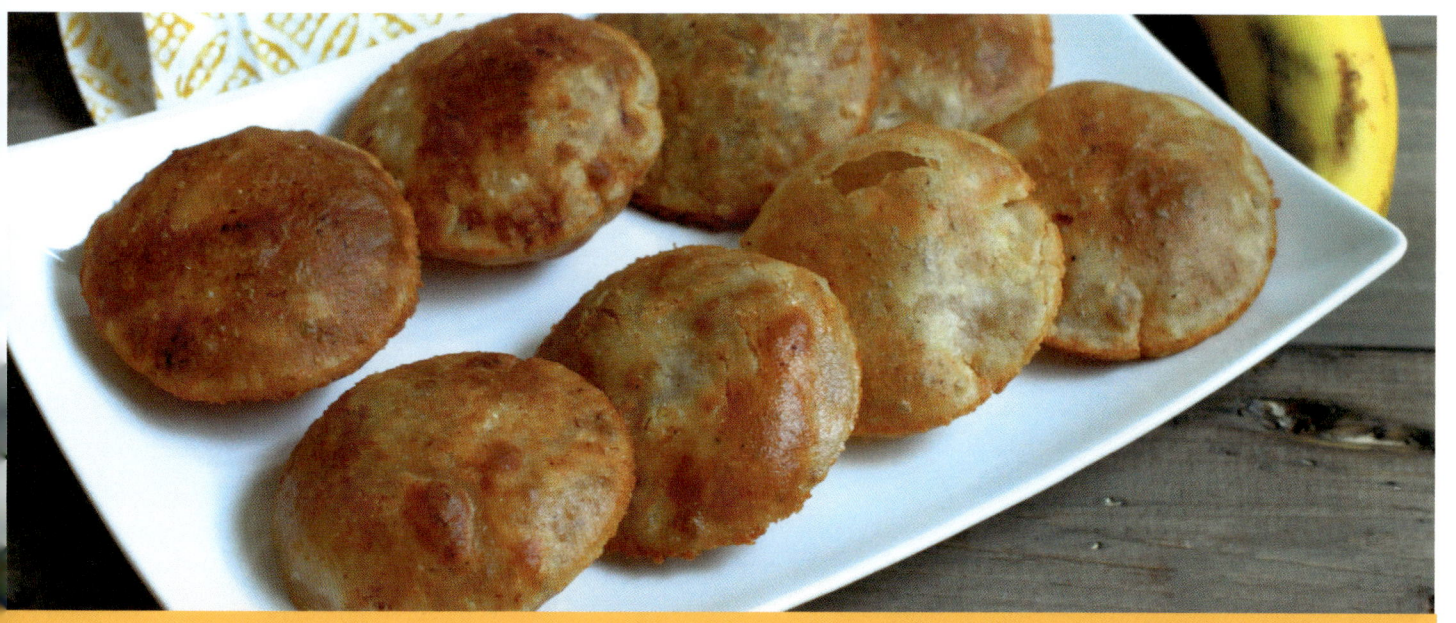

Banana Puri

Serves: 6-8   Time: 45 minutes

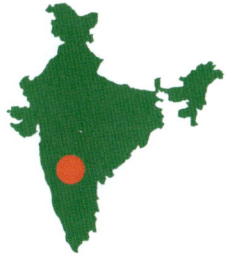

Ingredients:

- 1 cup cassava flour
- 1 ripe banana - medium sized - mashed
- 1 TBSP coconut oil
- pinch of pink salt
- 1/8 tsp cinnamon powder
- 2.5-3 TBSP water
- coconut or avocado oil for deep frying

Reintroduction Note:
If you've reintroduced cardamon, include 1/8 tsp with the cinnamon.

Method:

- Combine all the ingredients (except water and frying oil) in a large deep bowl
- Add water starting with 2 TBSP and up to 3 TBSP and knead until a stiff dough is formed. The amount of water needed will depend on the size of your banana.
- To knead the dough you'll need to work with your hands and keep working in the crumbs until a solid dough ball is formed
- Cover dough with a damp paper towel and put a plate over the bowl. Allow dough to set for 15 minutes.
- Divide the dough into 20 equal portions and roll into balls
- Roll each ball into a 2.5 inch circle by placing between 2 pieces of parchment paper .... *for perfecting round puri (which helps them to puff up nicely), use the top of a glass or a cookie cutter*
- Heat oil (coconut or avocado) in a deep pan over medium heat. You need at least 2-3 inches of oil in the pot to fry all the puri.
- Test the oil by dropping in a small piece of dough. It should bubble all around and start to float to the surface. Oil should have ripples on the surface, but stay below the smoking point.
- Place one puri in the oil and press lightly around the edges with a slotted spoon as puri begins to puff up.
- Allow to fry on first side for about 45 seconds until it starts to brown around the edges and puffs up.
- Flip and allow to cook on other side for about 45 seconds.
- *You'll need to experiment with your stove/ oil temperature/ cooking time to find what works best for you. On my stove I went back and forth between low & medium heat and was able to put a 2nd puri in the oil after flipping the first.*
- Remove from heat to plate with a paper towel to absorb excess oil
- Serve hot with a cup of kahwa (pg. 94).

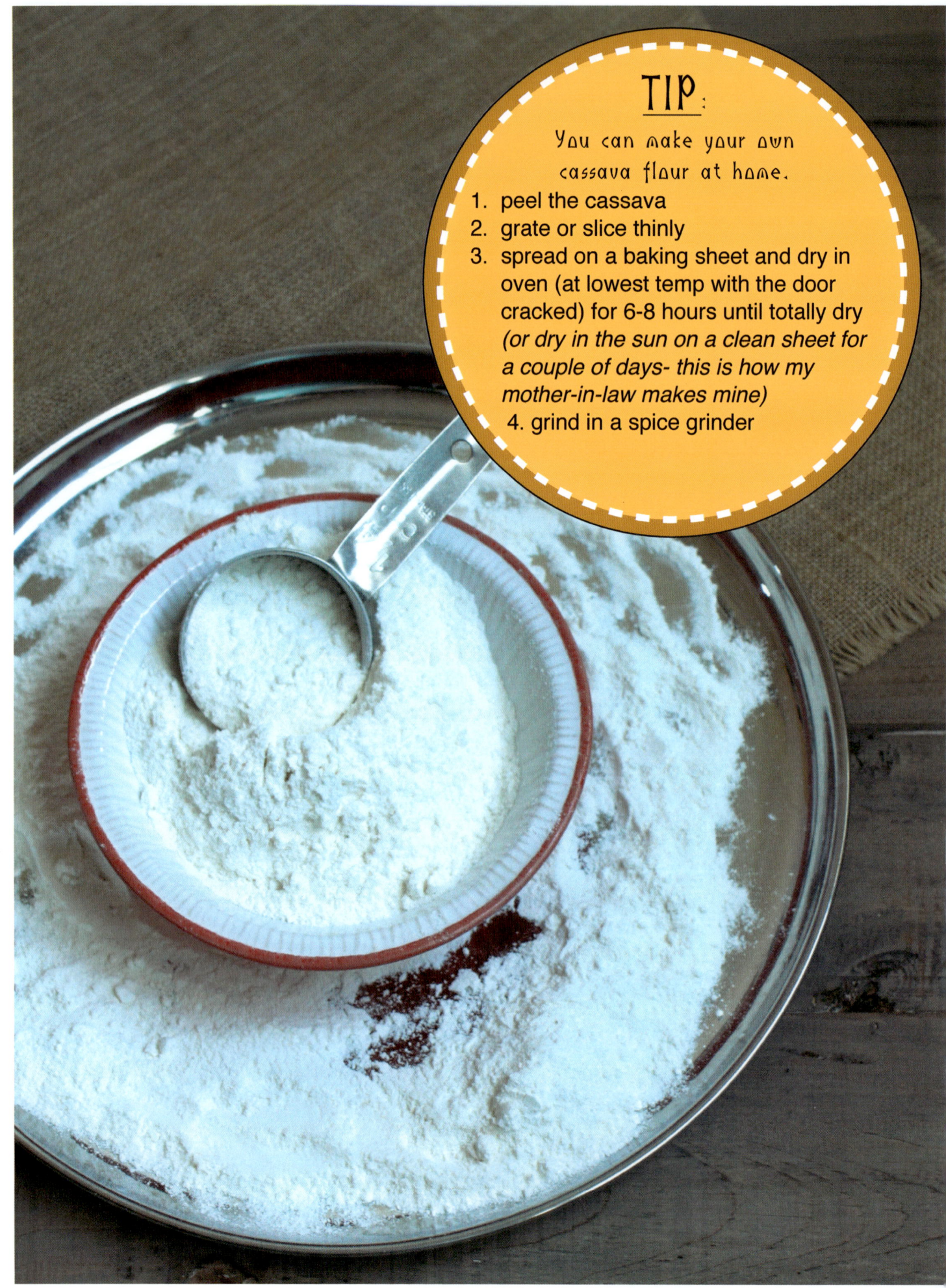

TIP:

You can make your own cassava flour at home.

1. peel the cassava
2. grate or slice thinly
3. spread on a baking sheet and dry in oven (at lowest temp with the door cracked) for 6-8 hours until totally dry *(or dry in the sun on a clean sheet for a couple of days- this is how my mother-in-law makes mine)*
4. grind in a spice grinder

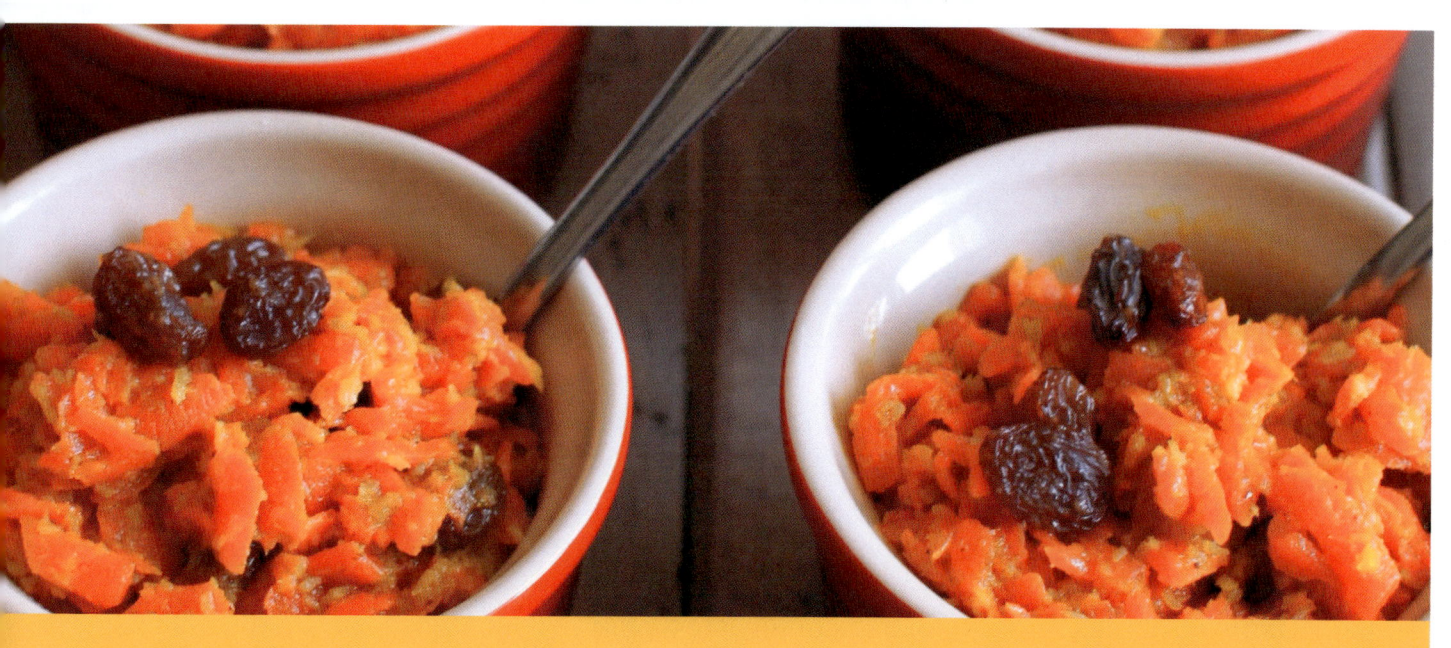

Carrot Halwa

Serves: 4   Time: 50 minutes

Ingredients:

- 3 cloves
- 1/8 tsp cinnamon powder
- 1/8 tsp ginger powder
- 2 TBSP coconut oil
- 2 1/2 cups grated carrots (about 4 large)
- 1 1/2 cups coconut milk
- 1/4 cup shredded coconut
- 3 TBSP coconut sugar
- 1/4 tsp pink salt
- 1/4 cup raisins
- *OPTIONAL - nuts for garnish (AIP reintroduction)*

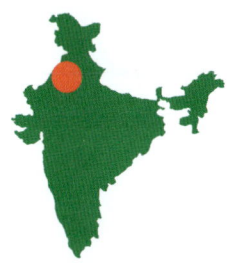

Method:

- wash, peel and grate the carrots - this is best done by hand
- heat a medium saucepan over a low to medium flame and add the spices to the dry pan - cloves, cinnamon & ginger and allow to dry roast until fragrant - about 90 seconds
- add coconut oil to pan and mix into spices and continue cooking about 30 seconds
- add grated carrots and stir well to incorporate oil and spices through the carrots
- let cook and start to soften for about 5 minutes
- add coconut milk and stir regularly until milk is more than half absorbed. This will take 15-20 minutes
- add coconut sugar, shredded coconut and salt and stir regularly until liquid is almost completely absorbed - no need to stir continually, just every 1-2 minutes. You may need to turn the heat down if the mixture starts to stick to the pan.
- add raisins and continue cooking and stirring continually until all liquid is absorbed.
- remove from heat and try to find the cloves and remove
- serve warm or cold - *optionally you can garnish with nuts (if you have reintroduced them.*

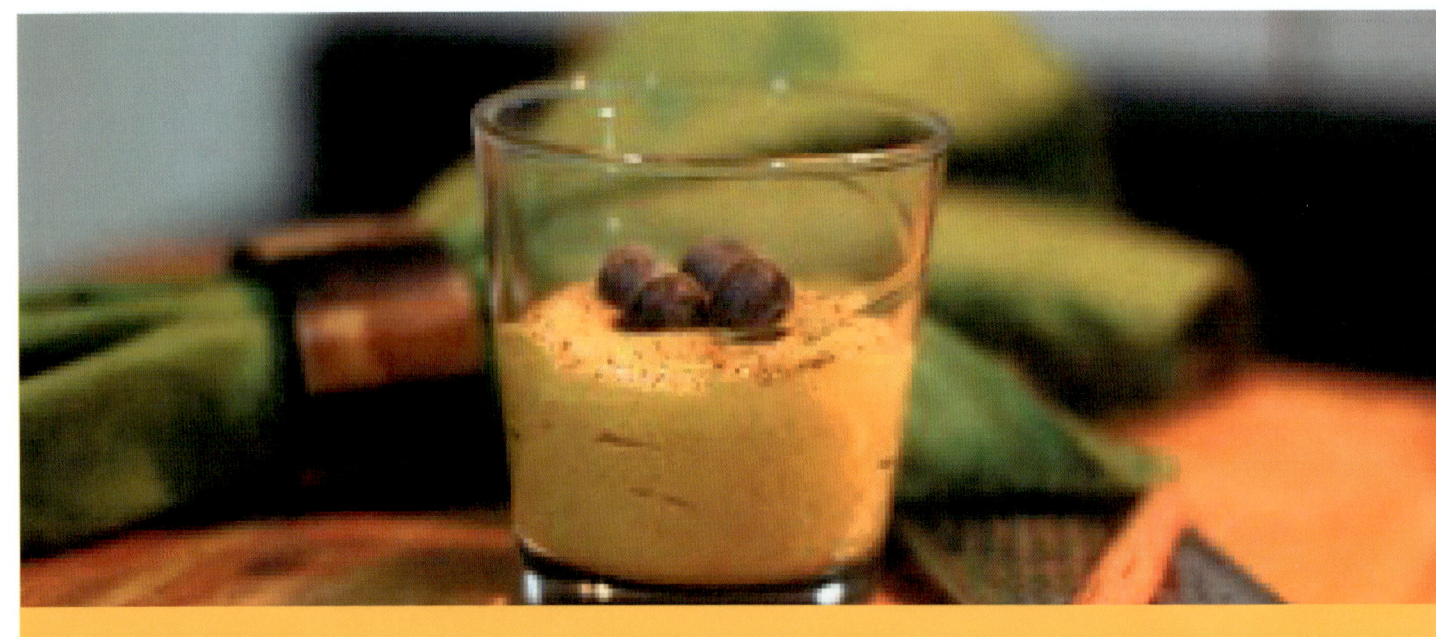

Saffron Mango Shrikhand

Serves: 2-3   Time: 5 minutes

Ingredients:
- 2 mangoes (divided)
- 1/2 can of good quality full fat coconut milk
- 5 dates – pitted
- a pinch of saffron threads
- 1/8 tsp cinnamon
- TOPPINGS - 1/4 cup toasted coconut & 1/2 mango chopped... or other fruits of choice (like blueberries)

Method:
- peel and dice the mangoes
- remove pits and soak dates in warm water for 5 minutes, then drain water
- place 1 1/2 mangoes and remaining ingredients in blender and blend until smooth
- mixture should be quite thick and creamy
- pour into serving dishes and place in the fridge to chill – after an hour it's thicker *and even better over night*
- right before serving, top with remaining mango and toasted coconut and/ or other fruits of choice

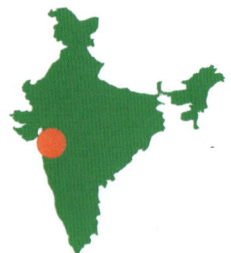

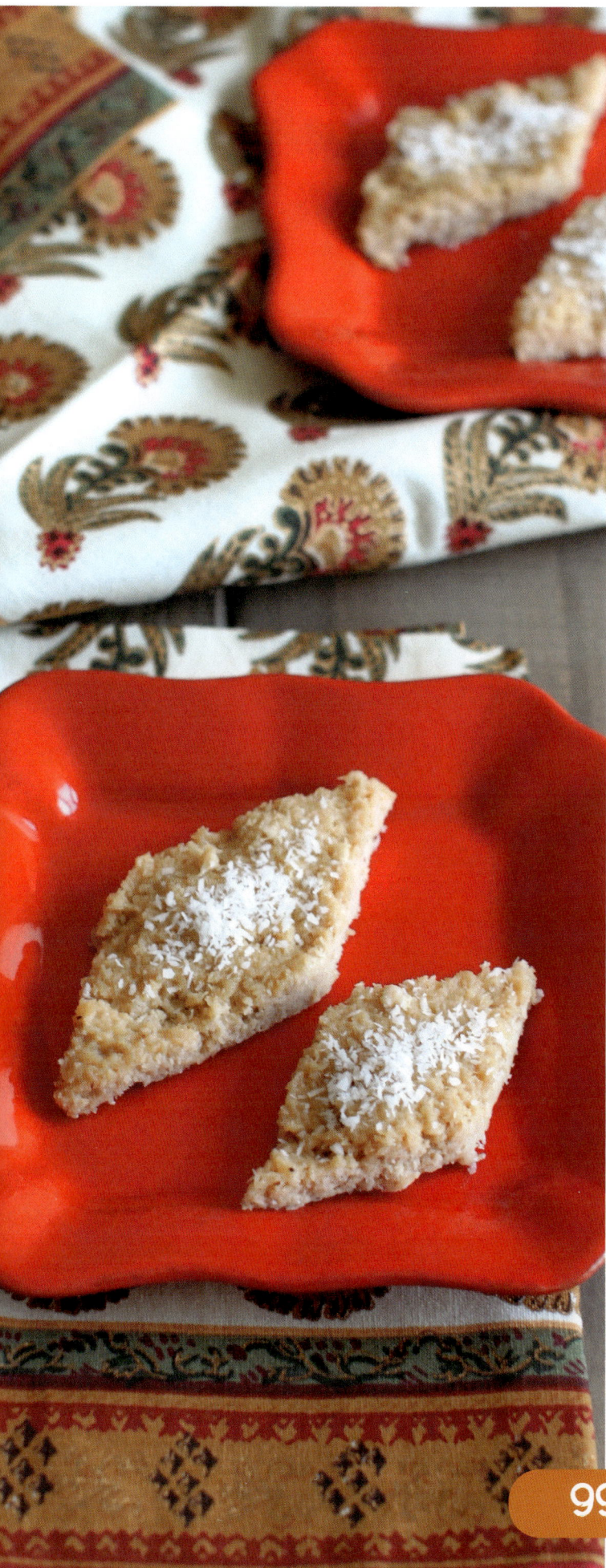

Coconut Burfi

Serves: 6   Time: 2 hours

Ingredients:
- 1 cup of coconut milk (canned or fresh)
- 1 cup unsweetened shredded coconut
- 1/4 cup coconut sugar
- 1/8 tsp ginger
- sprinkle of cinnamon & mace
- 1/4 cup water
- 3 TBSP coconut oil

Method:
- place all ingredients except coconut oil in medium saucepan over medium heat and bring to a low boil
- reduce to simmer over low heat and allow coconut mixture to cook for about 25 minutes stirring regularly (every minute or so)
- once much of the liquid has cooked off and mixture starts to form a ball when stirred, add 2 1/2 TBSP coconut oil and allow to keep cooking over low heat and stirring (about 10-15 minutes)
- once all liquid has cooked off and mixture resembles "wet sand" remove from the heat
- Use 1/2 TBSP coconut oil to grease an 8 x 8 pan and pour coconut mixture into the pan and smooth the top with the back of a spoon
- allow to cool on the counter for 20 minutes then score/ cut into pieces with a knife
- place in the freezer for another 20 minutes to harden before removing from the pan
- keep in the fridge for up to a week.

Reintroduction Note:
If you've reintroduced cardamon, include 1/8 tsp with the rest of the spices.

Ginger Mango Kulfi
with Toasted Coconut

Serves: 6   Time: 5 minutes

Ingredients:
- 2 mangos or 2 cups frozen mango
- 1/2 cup coconut cream
- 1 can coconut milk
- 1/2 tsp vanilla
- 1 TBSP ginger powder
- 1/4 cup honey
- 1/4 cup shredded coconut
- topping - toasted coconut - toast in dry pan for 1-2 minutes until golden

Method:
- cut mango
- mix all ingredients in a blender until creamy and smooth
- freeze overnight in popsicle molds or ramekins
- toast coconut in a dry pan over a medium heat for 1 minute until golden brown
- remove popsicles from molds and dip in coconut or remove from ramekins and top with toasted coconut

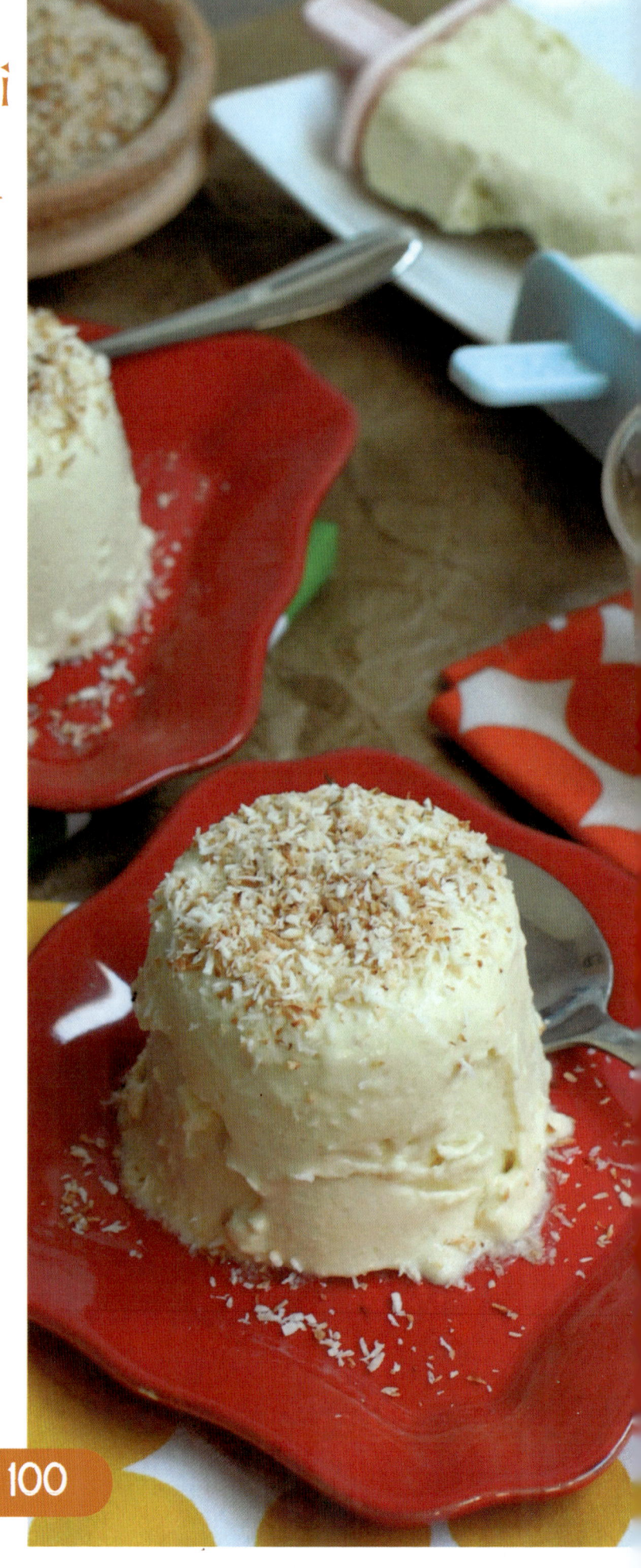

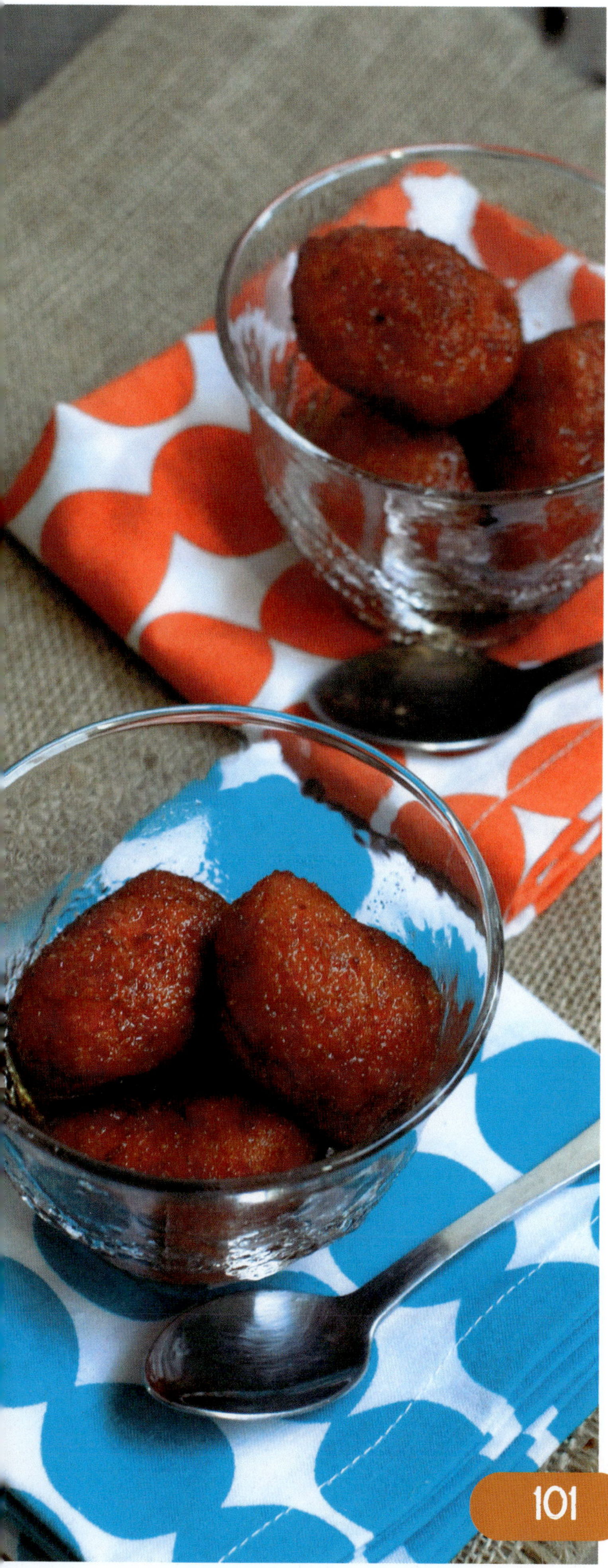

Sweet Potato Gulab Jamun

Serves: 5   Time: 2 hours

Ingredients:
- 1 large baked orange sweet potato (about 1.75 cup sweet potato puree)
- 1/2 cup cassava flour
- 1/4 tsp cinnamon
- 1/4 tsp pink himalayan salt
- 1/8 tsp baking soda
- oil for deep frying

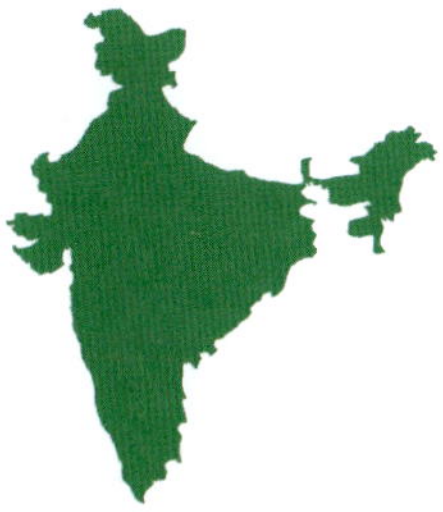

- 3 TBSP hot water
- 5 TBSP honey
- pinch of cinnamon, mace & cloves

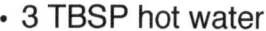

Method:
- cook sweet potato (microwave, bake or steam) - removed flesh from potato and mash well
- once potato has cooled, mix cassava flour, 1/4 tsp cinnamon, 1/4 tsp salt, 1/8 tsp baking soda until a dough is formed
- heat coconut or avocado oil in a saucepan on medium heat for deep frying - you want about 2-3 inches of oil
- use your hands to gently roll 16 balls - don't press hard on the dough or the gulab jamun will be hard - just gently roll between your hands - the dough will be sticky
- fry in batches (4-5 per batch) being careful not to overcrowd the pan - turn frequently while frying for a total of about 2.5-3 minutes until they turn golden brown and start to float
- remove from oil and place on plate lined with paper towel to cool
- make honey syrup - mix hot water (almost boiling), honey and pinch of cinnamon, mace and cloves and allow to cool a few minutes
- place cooled (room temp) gulab jamun into the syrup and allow to sit in syrup (turning occasionally) for 3 hours
- serve with a spoonful of syrup

Reintroduction Note:
Add pinch of cardamon to syrup as well.

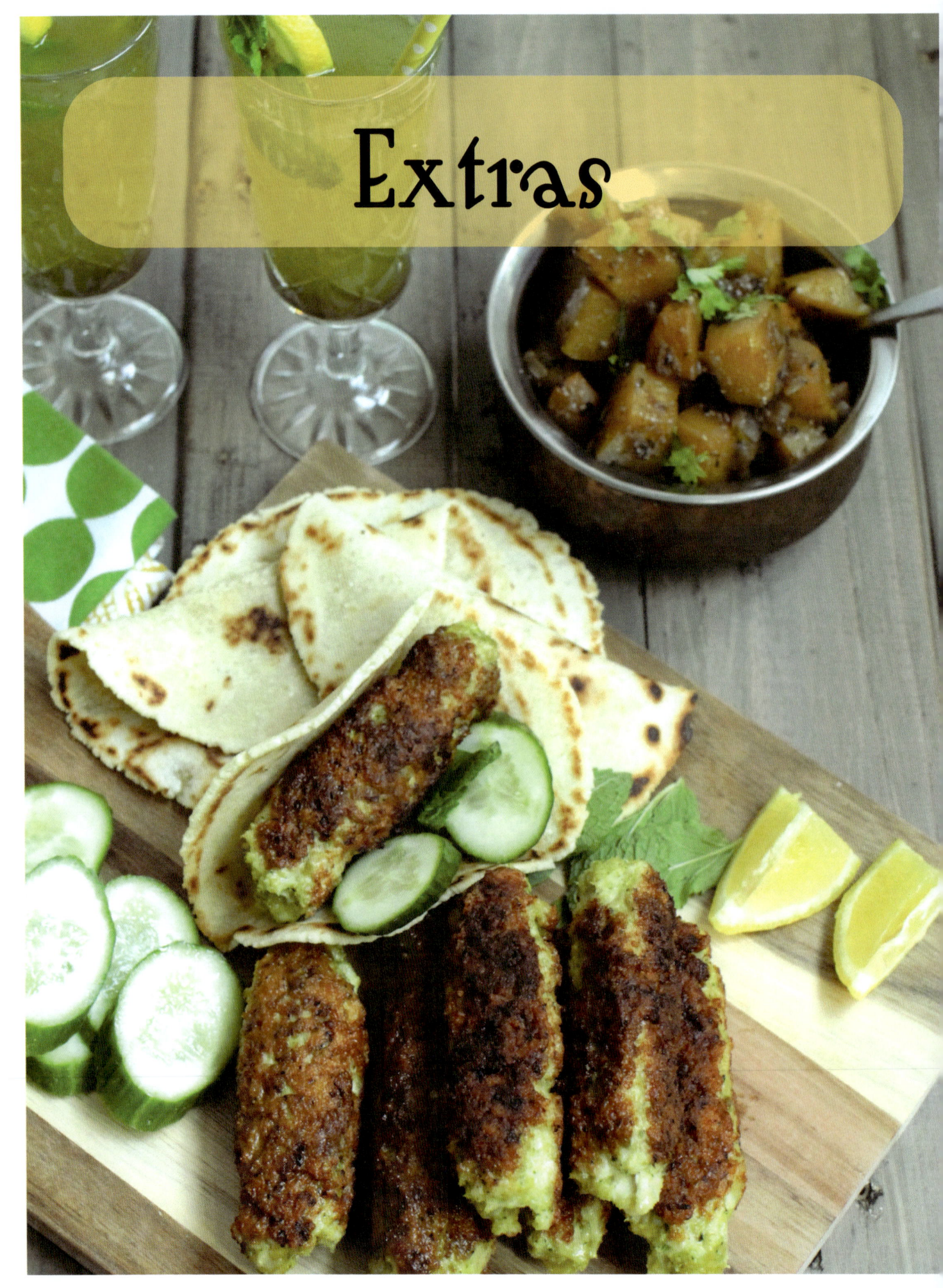

Extras

My AIP Indian Cooking Shopping List

Spices & Staples:

- Coconut Milk
- Coconut Cream
- Coconut Oil
- Shredded Coconut
- Coconut Sugar
- Coconut Flour
- Cassava Flour
- Tapioca Starch
- Ground Ginger
- Ground Cinnamon
- Cinnamon Sticks
- Ground Turmeric
- Garlic Powder
- Mace
- Saffron
- Cloves (whole & ground)
- Dried Curry Leaves
- Dried Fenugreek Leaves
- Dried Cilantro/ Coriander Leaf
- Sea Salt
- Pink Himalayan Salt
- Amchur Powder
- Dried Rose Petals
- Black Tea
- Green Tea
- Honey
- Tamarind

Produce:

- Fresh grated coconut
- Curry leaves
- Coriander leaves (cilantro)
- Fresh mint leaves
- Methi - fresh fenugreek
- Onions
- Fresh ginger
- Garlic
- Bitter Gourd
- Cabbage
- Carrots
- Cassava
- Cauliflower
- Mushrooms
- Okra
- Plantains
- Pumpkin
- Spinach
- Sweet Potatoes (white & orange)
- Banana
- Lemon
- Mangoes

Kitchen Tools:

- Blender or immersion blender
- Spice grinder or mortar & pestle
- Good knives and cutting boards
- Roti tawa - flat griddle pan for cooking roti and chapati
- Skewers
- Kulfi or popsicle molds

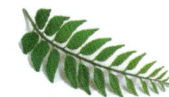

Frozen:

- Cassava pieces
- Mango pieces
- Frozen spinach

Coconut Free Recipes

Coconut Free Recipes & Recipe Substitutions

- Sweet Potato Paratha (use avocado oil instead of coconut oil)
- AIP Curry Powder
- Coconut Turmeric Rice (just omit the coconut)
- Coriander Chutney
- Mango Chutney (sub honey for coconut sugar & use olive oil)
- Date Tamarind Chutney (sub honey for coconut sugar))
- Plantain Bajis (fry in avocado oil)
- Kachumber Salad
- Onion Bajis (fry in avocado oil)
- Fish Cutlets (fry in olive oil)
- Turmeric Sweet Potatoes (fry in olive oil)
- Lamb Aloo Keema (omit the coconut milk)
- Lamb Biryani (marinate lamb in lemon juice instead of coconut milk)
- Spiced Lamb Kebabs (fry in olive oil)
- Curried Shepherd's Pie
- Prawn Masala
- Coriander Prawn Skewers
- Kerala Fried Fish (use olive oil for frying)
- Spicy Alu Makha
- Cabbage Thoran (omit the coconut)
- Cassava Thoran (omit the coconut)
- Simple Saag
- Aloo Gobi (use olive oil)
- Gajar Methi (sub honey for coconut sugar)
- Kaddu Ki Sabzi
- Chettinad Mushroom Masala (use olive oil)
- Spiced Bitter Gourd (replace coconut sugar with honey)
- Jal Jeera
- Rose Scented Iced Tea
- Thirst Quencher
- Kahwa
- Banana Puri
- Sweet Potato Gulab Jamun (use avocado oil for frying)

A Note on Reintroductions

The Autoimmune Protocol (AIP), at least in it's strictest sense, isn't meant to last forever. The idea behind AIP is that it's an elimination diet where you remove all potential inflammatory foods from your diet for a period and then you test foods one at a time to see if you can reintroduce them safely into your diet. Some people find they can start reintroductions after 30 days, some 90 days and for others it's years before they feel well enough to test foods.

How do you reintroduce:
1. Wait until your symptoms are in remission and you've given your gut time to heal. The length of time is different for everyone depending on your diagnosis and the extent of your disease progression.
2. Start with the least inflammatory foods and try one food at a time every 4-7 days and test the results. See the list below for the safest order for food reintroductions.
3. On the first day of the trial, eat a small bite of the food and see how you feel. Later in the day, eat another bite of the food and see how you feel.
4. The next day, eat a full serving of the food and see how you feel. If no symptoms return, try the same food again the 3rd day and rejoice that you have successfully reintroduced it.
5. If any symptoms return, put this food on the "NO" list and try again in a month or so if you want. Symptoms that might mean you're not tolerating the food are any of the symptoms of your autoimmune condition, bloating or any other gastrointestinal issues, headaches, anxiety, joint inflammation, or anything else that doesn't feel "right."
6. Wait a day and start the process again for the next food on your list.

Stage 1	Stage 2	Stage 3	Stage 4
- Berry spices (black pepper) - Egg yolks - Seed based spices (cumin, mustard, etc.) - Edible pod legumes (green beans, snow peas) - Ghee - Seed and nut oils	- Grass-fed butter - Egg whites - Cocoa - Alcohol (small amounts) - Nuts & Seeds (except pistachios & cashews)	- Coffee - Grass-fed cream and yogurt - Pistachios & cashews - Mild nightshades (paprika, eggplant)	- Other grass-fed dairy products - Other legumes - White rice - Alcohol (in moderation) - Other nightshades (potatoes, tomatoes and chili peppers)

Based on information in "The Paleo Approach" by Sarah Ballantyne, PhD.

For more detailed information on the reintroduction process, check out the book on AIP reintroductions by Eileen Laird of the Phoenix Helix.

Printed in Great Britain
by Amazon